Neurology Review
for the
NON-NEUROLOGIST

Rediscovering Neurology

HARVEY CASTRO, MD

Edited by Trisha Sheffield.

Cataloging-in-publication data is on file for this title at the Library of Congress.

Library of Congress Control Number: 2008904620

TABLE OF CONTENTS

Disclaimer: Medicine is a constantly changing science with research yielding new drug treatment and understanding of disease. Therefore, it is important to stay up to date and research the latest discoveries. The author, editor, and publisher have all made best efforts to provide information that is up-to-date, accurate, and generally accepted by medical standards at the time of publication. However, human error is always a possibility. The author, editor, and Publication Company involved with this printing do not warrant the information in this book as accurate or complete, nor are they responsible for omissions or errors in the book or for the results of use. It is the reader's responsibility to confirm information with other sources prior to use, specifically as it relates to all medications or treatment plans as these often change. It is important to read packet inserts and keep up with current doses and black box warnings from the FDA. Medicine is changing rapidly, and the print version of the book is not able to keep up with daily changes.

The idea for this book came to me during morning rounds when I was a medical student. I thought it would be great if I had a book that I could keep in one of my lab coat pockets as an easy reference to look up quick differentials and go over neurologic exams. I started reviewing different textbooks and adding pearls to each section of the neuro-exam. The book's format is set up as if you were doing a neurological exam and includes a differentials diagnosis in each topic. It is a great review for medical students, residents, or physicians who dislike reading neurology but need a quick review of the major high points. As an Emergency Medicine Physician, it has been a great review. I have also included "zebras" for those of us who want to show off at cocktail parties.

Regardless of outcome, you continue to be my biggest fan. I dedicate this book to you, to my mother and my children children Harvey, Zachary, Lauren, and Hailey.

I truly believe that everything is possible as long as you believe in yourself. Also, I would like to thank my mother Nydia Garcia for all her hard work and daily prayers. Finally, thanks to the following reviewers: Jeffery Gould MD, Luis Albuerne MD, and Payman Zamiour MD.. I also would like to thank Trisha Sheffield for her editorial assistance.

Remember that the eyes do not see what the mind does not know. Thank you for purchasing this book. If you have any comments or would like to contribute to the next edition.

ABBREVIATIONS:

CN: Cranial Nerves

ddx: Differential diagnosis

DM: Diabetes mellitus

Dx: Diagnosis

Rx: Treatment

S/s: Signs & symptoms

SE: Side Effect

Pt: Patient

(Z): Zebras

Neurology Review for the Non-Neurologist DPS 1st edition.

Harvey Castro, MD

NOTE: IT IS GOAL OF THE AUTHORS TO INDICATE STATE OF THE ART TREATMENTS FOR NOTED ILLNESSES. MEDICATIONS SUGGESTED FOR THE TREATMENT OF MEDICAL CONDITIONS MAY NOT BE FDA APPROVED FOR THE PURPOSE LISTED.

CRANIAL NERVES I-XII

Cranial Nerves (CN) I: Olfactory nerve exits the brain through the cribriform plate. It contains sensory nerve function;
Test for smell using non-noxious substance (coffee, cinnamon) by occluding one nostril, close the eyes, sniff, and ask if patient can smell.
Anosmia ddx: head injury, Neurosyphilis, mass lesion, Kallmann Syndrome, Zinc deficiency, Vitamin A deficiency, Multiple Sclerosis, and Refsum disease.
Zebra (Z): Kallmann Syndrome: anosmia, hypogonadotropic (decrease GnRH), and hypogonadism.
Dysosmia: distorted sense of smell.
Unilateral anosmia ddx: trauma; tumor.

CN II: Optic nerve passes the optic canal, sensory nerve responsible for sight;

Test: visual acuity, visual field, light reflex, accommodation, and fundus exam.

CN II Sites of lesion:

1. **Optic nerve**: Ipsilateral monocular loss of vision.
    ddx: trauma, vasculitis, tumor, and optic neuritis.

2. **Optic chiasm**:
    *   **Midsagittal transection or pressure**: Bitemporal hemianopsia. **ddx**: pituitary adenoma, pituitary apoplexy, and craniopharyngioma.
    *   **Bilateral compression**: Binasal hemianopsia. **ddx**: calcified internal carotids.

3. **Optic tract**: Homonymous hemianopsia.
    ddx: abscess or tumor of temporal lobe.

4. **Optic radiations***:*
    *   **Temporal lobe or Meyers loop**: Superior homonymous quadrantanopsia, "pie in the sky."
    *   **Parietal lobe**: Inferior homonymous quadrantanopsia.
    *   **Geniculate body**: Homonymous hemianopsia.
        ddx: AVM, and infarction.

5. **Occipital lobe**: Variable ocular manifestations of systemic disease. (Commonly: homonymous hemianopsia with macular sparing.)
    ddx: PCA stroke, and neoplasm.

(Z): **Methanol Poisoning**: Causes optic nerve blindness, and papillitis due to the metabolic byproduct (formaldehyde). Pt complains of "looking into a snowstorm." Other symptoms include seizures, headaches appearing 12-18 hrs later.

Labs: Increase anion gap metabolic acidosis.

Rx: Fomepizole, or ETOH, sodium bicarbonate.

Other lesions to eye:

1. **Conjunctivitis in newborn:** If within the first 24hrs, chemical conjunctivitis is likely to be the cause; if later then G/C (Gonorrhea 3-7 days & Chlamydia 7-14 days), infection should be ruled out.

2. **Herpes Simplex Keratitis:** Dendritic corneal ulcers lesions seen
with fluorescein.
Rx: Idoxuridine.

3. **Iritis ddx**: Ankylosing spondylitis, Reiter syndrome, and Behcet
disease.
ddx: Acute vision loss: retinal detachment status post trauma, or eye surgery. Thoracic Aortic Dissection (especially with chest pain)
S/s: Complain of seeing "flashes or floaters" or loss of part of visual field; Patients with myopia are at increase risks.
Dx: by indirect ophthalmoscope evaluation.
Rx: This situation is considered an emergency referral.

4. **Retinal artery occlusion:** Symptoms include abrupt, painless almost complete unilateral visual loss, 2nd to emboli originating from carotid artery disease or valvular heart disease.
S/s: Classic findings fixed dilated pupil, cherry red spot (if the entire central retinal artery is occluded) and diffuse retinal whitening. "Amaurosis fugax" may suggest giant cell arteritis.
Rx: ocular massage or carbogen therapy (breathing into a paper bag causes vasodilation) & carbonic anhydrase

inhibitors. Emergency referral to an ophthalmologist (anterior chamber paracentesis) with a work up towards the cause of the event. This may include a stroke workup since most patients have a significant systemic disease (DM & hypertension) and cardiovascular risk factors.

5. **Retinal vein occlusion**:
   S/s: gradual painless vision loss. Extensive retinal hemorrhages, dilated & tortuous retinal veins, edematous, and congested fundus. **ddx**: hypertension, DM, trauma, tumor, & hypercoagulability state.
   Rx: emergency ophthalmologic consult.

6. **ddx for cherry red spot on macula: central artery occlusion,** Tay Sachs & Niemann Picks.

7. **Niemann-Pick disease:** Sphingomyelinase deficiency on chromosome 11, foamy histocytes in liver, spleen (hepatosplenomegaly), anemia, and neurologic deficit. Type A is fatal in kids. Type B can survive to adulthood.

8. **Tay Sachs:** Hexosaminidase A defect, mental retardation, blind with no hepatosplenomegaly.

9. **Anisocoria:** Unequal size of pupils, congenital or acquired.

10. **Aniridia:** Absence of the iris, associated with congenital abnormality such as Wilms tumor (Nephroblastoma).

11. **Adie's Pupil:** (idiopathic tonic pupil) "large & irregular." When light is shined on pupil, the pupil is slow to constrict or constricts incompletely then remains constricted for an abnormally long time. In early stages, the pupil is dilated. Accommodation is impaired along with constriction of the pupil. +/- impaired **D**eep **T**endon **R**eflexes (**DTR**). Typically seen in females, unilateral pupil (80%) of the time.

Dx: examine iris with slit lamp. Instillation of weak cholinergic agents (1/8% pilocarpine HCL) will cause constriction of tonic pupil because of denervation hypersensitivity.

12. **Argyll Robertson Pupil:** Pupil that accommodates to near objects but does not react to light. The pupil fails to dilate after atropine administration, associated with tertiary syphilis.
    Test: RPR & fluorescent treponemal antibody-absorption test.

13. **(Z): Cyanide poisoning:** Causes optic neuropathy
    Antidote - nitrite, hydroxocobalamin, and thiosulfate.

14. **Retinal Exam ddx**: "Arteriovenous nicking," "copper/silver wiring," Flame hemorrhages are retinal signs seen in hypertension, and artherosclerosis.

15. **Pediatrics:** If newborn has decreased red reflex or leukocoria (white pupil), should rule out: retinoblastoma or cataracts. If the infant is found to have cataracts then rule out galactosemia.

16. **Cotton Wool Exudates:** White, fuzzy areas on the surface of the retina caused by damage to retinal layer. Common signs of: DM, HTN, AIDS, collagen vascular disease, and SLE.

17. **Exophthalmos:** Protrusion of an eye globe. Causes include congenital, familial, retro-orbital tumor, thyroid disease. Hyperthyroidism and Graves' disease usually cause bilateral exophthalmus.

18. **Hollenhorst plaques**: Yellow cholesterol emboli in the retinal arterioles originate from carotid artery or great vessels.

19. **Horner syndrome**:
    S/s: miosis, ptosis, hemi anhidrosis, hyperemia, (apparent) enophthalmos, associated with Pancoast tumor that is usually located at the apex of lung or lesion in the hypothalamospinal tract above T1.

Dx: by phenylephrine 1 % in eye will cause miosis in Horner's syndrome but dilates eye in the normal patient. Consider CT scan of chest to rule out tumor.

20. **Ischemic optic neuropathy**: Sudden painless, unilateral visual loss, swollen disc, and arcuate field defect.

21. **Marcus Gunn Pupillary Sign:** Lesion is in the afferent portion of the light reflex. When light is shined on the diseased eye, pupil will dilate. Condition can be seen in optic neuritis, tumor, and glaucoma.

22. **Miosis ddx:** Pupillary diameter < 2 mm: PCP, opioids (most), organophosphates & cholinergics, phenothiazine, nicotine, pontine hemorrhage, & CNS infections (neurosyphilis).

23. **Mydriasis ddx**: Pupillary diameter > 6 mm: Sympathomimetics (cocaine), atropine, anticholinergics, phenytoin, cimetidine, antihistamines, barbiturates, withdrawal of substances of abuse, anoxia, CN III damage, thyrotoxicosis & acute angle glaucoma.

24. **Optic neuritis** (associated with Multiple Sclerosis)**:** Ocular pain with movement & afferent pupillary impairment.

25. **Extraocular muscles innervation**: **LR6SO4R3** Lateral **R**ectus CN 6, **S**uperior **O**blique CN 4, the **R**est of the eye muscles CN 3.

26. **Ptosis ddx**: Horner's, 3rd CN (diabetes mellitus, **T**rauma, **T**emporal lobe, orbital pseudo-**T**umor, **T**hyroid disease, Myasthenia gravis, & **T**rauma (blow out orbital fracture)/ previous eye surgery.

27. **Roth spots**: A round white retinal area surrounded by small hemorrhage associated with endocarditis.

CN III: Oculomotor passes through superior orbital fissure. Motor function: levator palpebrae (eyelid opening), upper eyelid, superior rectus, medial rectus, inferior rectus, inferior oblique muscle, parasympathetic fibers to sphincter muscles for iris pupil constriction & ciliary muscles for accommodation.

CN III lesion: Causes deviation downward, ptosis & external rotation, inability to rotate eye inward, non-responsive pupil dilated & cycloplegia (paralysis of accommodation). If there is complete paralysis of CN III, then the patient will have both horizontal & vertical diplopia.

CN III lesions common ddx: 3rd nerve palsy, intracranial aneurysm (posterior communicating artery), vaso-occlusive disease within nerve, hypertension, diabetes mellitus (pupil is not affected), syphilis, primary amyloidosis, polyarteritis nodosa, trauma, brain tumor & Myasthenia gravis.

(Z): Benedikt's (dorsal midbrain)**:** Hemiplegia with clonic spasm or intention tremor & CN III oculomotor paralysis on the opposite side. Causes include infarction, hemorrhage & tumor. (Combine Claude and Weber syndrome = Benedikt)

(Z): Claude's syndrome: CN III palsy, ipsilateral pupillary dilatation, diminished blinking, increased lacrimation with contralateral cerebellar ataxia & tremor. Physical findings are similar to Benedikt syndrome without the hemiparesis.

(Z): Weber syndrome (ventral midbrain): Paralysis of CN III, i.e. dilated eye, ptosis on one side & hemiplegia of opposite side (UMN), Causes include paramedian infarct of midbrain or impending uncal herniation.

CN IV: Trochlear nerve passes through superior orbital fissure. Motor function: eye movement is medially & inferior deviation.

CN IV lesion: Trochlear nerve; Superior oblique muscle causes vertical diplopia that worsens when looking down. Patient will have downgaze & tilts head to opposite shoulder to compensate for the diplopia. Classically, the patient will have trouble walking down stairs.
ddx: close head trauma, small vessel disease, hypertension, diabetes mellitus, tumor, Miller-Fisher variant of Guillain-Barre Syndrome, aneurysms & meningitis. In children, consider congenital or traumatic cause.

CN V: Trigeminal nerve from nucleus: Motor and sensory functions for the face. Motor: mastication (masseter, pterygoids & temporalis muscle); sensation: face and afferent limb of corneal reflex.
Check: facial sensation with cold and pin, corneal sensation (with gauze), & masseter strength. (V1) exits the skull through superior orbital fissure providing forehead sensation & corneal sensation and reflex. (V2) exits the foramen rotundum with function of infraorbital, palate & upper teeth sensation. (V3) exits foramen ovale allowing mandibular, chin, lower teeth & tongue sensation.
Trigeminal ganglion lesion: Motor and sensation dysfunction depending on specific location of injury in brainstem. The patient may have change of sensation in the neck and posterior aspect of head.

CN V lesion: Motor nerve: paralysis of tensor tympani: *hypo*acusis (decrease sound). Jaw deviates to side of lesion. Sensory lesion: decrease sensation of corresponding nerve. Decreased periocular sensation & decreased corneal sensation.

ddx: Trauma, Lyme, sarcoidosis, Sjögren's syndrome, trauma, arsenic poisoning & trigeminal neuralgia.

Sturge Weber: Port wine stain (nevus) extends over the sensory distribution of V1 V2, V3. Leptomeningeal vascular malformations with intracranial calcification occur on the same side as the port wine stain.
S/s: include contralateral focal seizures, hemiparesis, hemianopia, mental retardation & ipsilateral congenital glaucoma. Vascular malformation (choroid), CSF elevated protein, skull x-ray "tram track calcifications" or "serpentine" appearance.
Rx: anti-epileptics; laser dermatologic surgery.
(Z): If Port wine stain on midline of back, associated with AV malformations of spinal cord.

Trigeminal neuralgia (Tic douloureux): 40 y/o⁺, female>male, sudden, severe, short duration or persistent, unilateral pain; symptoms can be triggered by touching affected area or chewing. Disease can be associated with Multiple Sclerosis, vascular disease, & tumor in posterior fossa or 5th CN tumor.
Check: dental caries, MRI with & without contrast special attention to CN V.
Rx: carbamazepine, gabapentin, oxcarbazine, phenytoin, lamotrigine, baclofen, ETOH injection into the nerve, or surgery for refactory cases which may include decompression of CN V, gamma knife surgery.
ddx of facial pain: post-herpetic neuralgia, carotidynia, cluster headache & trigeminal neurologia.

CN VI: Abducens nerve passes through superior orbital fissure. Eye movement - abduction caused by lateral rectus muscle.

CN VI lesion: Abducens nerve: lateral rectus muscle. Paralysis, loss of abduction & horizontal diplopia, greatest separation of gaze directed toward affected side. Causes include intracranial tumors/pressure, isolated 6th CN damage, MS, stroke, neurosarcoidosis, and mass lesion.

Internuclear ophthalmoplegia (INO): Lesion to MLF (medical longitudinal fasciculus): carries CN 6 nucleus to contralateral 3rd medial rectus subnucleus, as a result failure of adduction in horizontal gaze but with retention of convergence. Exam demonstrates nystagmus of abducting eye in lateral gaze, uni (bi) lateral. In older patients, consider small vessel disease within vertebral basilar arterial system, diabetes mellitus(DM) & hypertension. In young adults consider demyelination disease (multiple sclerosis). In children, check for Pontine glioma & multiple sclerosis.

(Z): Parinaud's syndrome: Dorsal midbrain:
1. Impaired up gaze
2. Convergence refractory nystagmus on attempted upgaze.
3. Fixed pupils & eyelid retraction.

This disease is associated with germinoma, pinealoma & hydrocephalus.

CN VII: Facial nerve passes the internal auditory meatus. It controls facial movement, anterior 2/3 taste, lacrimation, salivation (submaxillary & submandibular salivary glands) & efferent limb of corneal reflex. On physical exam, ask patient to smile & inflate cheeks then squeeze eyes tightly, attempt to open eyes & say Mi, Mi... (check: lips)

Check: for loss of corneal reflex (efferent), must consider CN V lesion also causing this.

CN VII lesion: Motor: hyperacusis (stapedius paralysis). If lesion to CV VII nucleus, then weakness of the ipsilateral upper & lower face (LMN weakness), see corticobulbar tract. Diabetes mellitus (known or new diagnosis). Other conditions include Lyme disease, Mastoiditis, Porphyria & primary Amyloidosis.

Blepharospasm: Involuntary spasmodic contraction of the orbicularis oculi muscle.

Bells palsy: Unilateral facial weakness that involves forehead & lower face. Ipsilateral - sagging mouth angle causing drooling, no smile, hyperacusis, decrease taste of anterior 2/3 of tongue, & inability to wrinkling forehead symmetrically (LMN) *(Central lesions **do not** affect forehead muscles; peripheral lesions **do** affect forehead.)*. Patients with increase risks include: diabetics, pregnant & females.
Rx: Increasing dose of corticosteroids decreases disease course. Do not use if suspect Lyme disease. It is important to give eye patch & wetting drops to prevent keratitis. Use acyclovir if herpes is suspected.

Chvostek's Sign: Facial irritability: unilateral spasm of the orbicularis oculi/oris muscle being induced by taping over the facial nerve.
Check: for hypocalcemia, ionized calcium levels; give calcium gluconate slowly.
(Z): Guillain-Barré syndrome, **Crocodile tears:** tearing unilateral when chewing; CN 7 regrows towards lacrimal gland instead of salivary gland.

Other causes of Facial Paresis:

1. Progressive weakness of one side of face with no sensory loss should suspect sarcoidosis.

2. If the patient is an infant, then should suspect neuropathy caused by delivery.

3. Sickle cell crisis, trauma, s/p parotidectomy.

(Z): Möbius syndrome: Congenital facial diplegia (CN VII) can be partial or complete facial nerve palsy & convergent strabismus (VI); eye sensitivity due to inability to squint.

Ramsay-hunt: Facial paralysis, otalgia, & herpes zoster resulting from viral infection of the 7th CN, and geniculate ganglion; vertigo, ipsilateral hearing deficit, & facial palsy plus vesicles in the external auditory canal. *Tzanck* smear positive.
Rx: acyclovir or famcyclovir & prednisone. Prednisone use always coupled with H2 blocker. The use of prednisone is controversial, probably not of benefit greater than seven days after onset or when known etiology (Diabetes, etc.).

CN VIII: Vestibulocochlear nerve exits skull through the internal auditory meatus: hearing, balance.
Check: Vestibular: gaze nystagmus, caloric testing, past pointing, and marching in place.
Check: Cochlear nerve: rub fingers together with patient's eyes closed on each side to see if patient can hear to same degree; Weber & Rinne tests to diagnose side of injury.

Balance consists of:
1. Dorsal column
2. Visual component.
3. Vestibular-midline cerebellum.

Caloric stimulation (Vestibular caloric test): First, verify that the patient has an intact eardrum. The next step is to injection water into the external auditory canal. Remember **COWS**: **C**OLD water causes the fast component of nystagmus toward the **O**PPOSITE side. Mechanism is that the corrective action is by the cortex and is fast. **W**ARM stimulation then the fast component of the nystagmus will be towards the **S**AME side. If the labyrinth is diseased or nonfunctional, there may be diminished or absent nystagmus. In a comatose patient with cerebral damage, the fast phase of the nystagmus will be absent. If both fast and slow are absent then this suggestions the patients brainstem reflexes are damaged.

Nystagmus: Involuntary rhythmic oscillation of the eyeballs, vertigal, horizontal, rotary, combination with a slow and fast component. This may be congenital.

Three types of benign nystagmus:
1. **End gaze** nystagmus - patient attempts to keep eyes at extremes of lateral gaze. Eyes will drift back slightly then re-fixate with small jerk movements.
2. **Drugs**: diphenylhydantoin, barbiturates & other sedatives.
3. **Searching**, pendular nystagmus: most positions of gaze have oscillations equal in speed & amplitude, usually arising from a visual disturbance from congenital, multiple sclerosis & vascular disease.

Vestibular Nystagmus: Due to labyrinth or nerve tracks. Labyrinthine component patient will have a horizontal & rotary component: slow phase to side of lesion. Peripheral causes horizontal nystagmus or rotary; the fast component will be opposite the lesion; central nystagmus causes vertical nystagmus.

Down beat Nystagmus: Nystagmus with the fast phase beating in a downward direction. This can be indicative of lesions from the foramen magnum, Chiari malformation, Wernicke disease & lithium toxicity.

Up beat Nystagmus: Caused from cerebellar lesion, BPPV, brainstem, multiple sclerosis & alcoholic cerebellar degeneration.

Horizontal Nystagmus: Ataxic nystagmus causes include internuclear ophthalmoplegia, multiple sclerosis & stroke**.**

See-Saw Nystagmus: Typical in chiasmal lesions.

Cerebellar lesion: Nystagmus: most of the time the fast component of the nystagmus is towards lesion.

CN **VIII lesion**:

Acoustic neuroma: (acoustic schwannoma)
   S/s: unilateral hearing loss, tinnitus, not debilitating dizziness/ vertigal, vestibular schwannoma invade cerebellar or brainstem. **Test:** MRI with gad or CT scan with special attention to CN VIII; 90 % of cerebello-pontine angle (CPA) tumors are acoustic neuromas. If bilateral, suspect: **Neurofibromatosis II** (NF2 gene). **Rx:** surgery, radiation therapy, & observation.

ddx of sudden deafness: Trauma, infectious (mumps, influenza, varicella, and mononucleosis), conductive (cerumen, OM, OE), & drug induced (aminoglycoside).

(Z): Alport syndrome: (sounds like airport) Deafness, hereditary nephritis, and sensory neurologic deficit (VIII), & ophthalmologic complications (lens dislocation); X-linked collagen defect.

Vertigo: Central vs. Peripheral:

- **Central vertigo**: has an insidious onset with vertical nystagmus not inhibited by ocular fixation; may have other CN or neurological abnormalities, normal caloric test, not positional related, no tinnitus.
  ddx: stroke, multiple sclerosis, CN VIII lesion & vertebrobasilar ischemia.

- **Peripheral vertigo**: abrupt onset, horizontal nystagmus improved with ocular fixation and complete head stillness, otherwise CN normal, abnormal caloric test, tinnitus, nausea, vomiting, hearing loss +/-, positional related. Condition is usually seen in younger patients.
  ddx: BPPV, Ménière disease, motion sickness, vestibular neuritis & acoustic neuromas.

Vertigo: Sensation of abnormal movements of the body or surroundings.
Acute vertigo ddx: Toxic damage to labyrinth, Trauma, Tumor, vertebrobasilar stroke & cerebellar hemorrhage.
Recurrent vertigo ddx: Meniere, Migraine & Multiple sclerosis.
Positional: BPPV, cervical, central & postinfectious.

Anti-vertiginous medications & SE:
1. **Meclizine** (Antivert) **SE**: drowsiness, ↑ bronchial secretions
2. **Dimenhydrinate** (Dramamine) **SE**: blurred vision, hallucinations, may worsen narrow angle glaucoma.
3. **Scopolamine: SE**: blurred vision.
4. **Valium:** drowsiness (use sparingly)

Antiemetics:
1. **Promethazine** (Phenergan) **SE**: extrapyramidal signs (acute

dystonic reactions), hypotension & dry mouth.

2. **Prochlorperazine** (Compazine) **SE**: extrapyramidal signs, & hypotension.

Benign paroxysmal positional vertigo (**BPPV**): Elderly, paroxysmal vertigo lasts seconds to minutes; horizontal nystagmus that occurs in certain critical head positions; no associated hearing loss or tinnitus. **Dx:** Dix-Hallpike test, MRI: R/o cerebellopontine angle lesion.

Rx: give antiemetics (Promethazine) 30 min prior to Epley maneuver reposition of displaced remnants of utricular otoconia (calcium carbonate crystals), 90% successful.

Labyrinthitis: Acute onset of vertigo that worsens with head movement. Other symptoms include fluctuating hearing loss, nystagmus, & tinnitus. Auditory or neurologic signs & symptoms depend on cause of labyrinthitis. Vertigo can last for days.

The **ddx** includes physiologic, infection (viral), drug induced, tumor, idiopathic being most common cause. If the origin is physiologic or emotional, then hyperventilate patient to replicate symptoms.

Rx: The disease is short-lived and self-limited. Can use **Meclizine**.

NOTE: Hearing loss does not occur with benign paroxysmal vertigo & vestibular neuronitis but occurs with infectious labyrinthitis and Ménière disease.

Ménière's Disease: Endolymphatic hydrops: recurrent attacks, older patients, remember Ménière's triad:

1. Sudden severe vertigal (lasting hours to days).
2. Fluctuating tinnitus
3. "Deafness" with N/V, horizontal nystagmus. Patients will demonstrate past pointing & falling to the side of the affected

ear. + Abnormal audiogram & Bárány sign negative.

Rx:
1. **Antihistaminic** agents **Dimenhydrinate** (Dramamine) SE: hallucinations, dry mouth & psychosis.
2. **Meclizine** (Antivert) Side effect: glaucoma.
3. **Chronic Rx:** decrease Na^{++} (diet of 1500 mg/day), diuretics (Acetazolamide SE: metabolic acidosis, tinnitus).

Hallpike maneuver or Bárány maneuver: Patient begins at the sitting position then is rapidly brought to the supine position. The next step is to quickly turn the head to one side. Observe for nystagmus & vertigo; repeat test towards the other side.

Other causes of lesions to VIII: Aspirin, Aminoglycoside, Neomycin, Ethacrynic acid, infection, stroke, sarcoidosis, Wegner's Granulomatosis, & meningitis.

Presbycusis: Usually in the elderly, decrease speech discrimination, hypersensitivity to noise, first affects the highest sound frequencies (18 to 20 kHz).

Rinne's test: Tuning fork is placed on mastoid process (tests bone conduction). As soon as the sound ceases, it is held by the auditory meatus (air conduction). This test compares bone conduction to air conduction. With middle ear loss of conduction, the air sound will not be appreciated after bone conduction, i.e loudest on mastoid (Rinne -). In nerve damage, the reverse is true (Rinne +). In summary, in conductive hearing loss, the Rinne test is negative & Weber test demonstrates lateralization to that side. In sensorineural hearing loss, the Weber test lateralizes to the ear and the Rinne test is positive.

Schwabach test: Comparing the patient's bone conduction with a normal examiner. In sensorineural loss, the patient stops hearing before the examiner. In conductive loss, the patient hears it longer than the examiner. The examiner must have normal hearing.

Weber test: 512 Hz tuning fork is placed on top of head; the test distinguishes between unilateral sensory & conduction loss. In a normal patient, the sound is appreciated equally on both sides. The sound will lateralize louder to side of conductive loss, but in nerve deafness, the sound will lateralize to the normal ear. In summary, if there is no localization, then this is normal for this test. If it localizes to the nonsymptomatic ear, then think of sensorineural cause. If it localizes to the symptomatic ear, then think of a conduction cause. If the patient has a sensorineural deficits bilateral (noise, ototoxicity) then both Weber & Rinne will be normal with diminished hearing.

Conductive hearing loss ddx: Foreign body (esp. in kids), wax, infection, & tumor.

Sensorineural hearing loss ddx: Drug induced (aminogylcosides), Labrinthis, viral neuritis, Acoustic Neuroma, & Congenital.

Syncope: Loss of consciousness and postural tone with spontaneous recovery. Must check orthostatic changes (laying, sitting, standing) in all patients with this problem.

Syncope ddx: Cardiac (vasovagal, orthostatic, arrhythmia, valvular) 90% of all syncope; Postmicturition syncope; drug-induced syncope (impair autonomic reflex mechanisms); metabolic (hypoglycemia, hypoxia, hypokalemia); psychiatry (hyperventilation hypocapnia); subclavian steal syndrome;

hypovolemia; & neurologic disorders (cerebral ischemia & seizures).

Drug-induced syncope: Diuretics, antihypertensives, & tricyclic medications.

Orthostatic hypotension: Reflex vasoconstriction & increase in heart rate with a fall in BP (typically > 20/10 mm Hg) on assuming a more upright posture. Orthostatic hypotension is not a specific disease but a manifestation of abnormal blood pressures due to many different causes which can be divided into 2 large categories:
1. **Non-neurogenic:** cardiac, medication induced, reduced intravascular volume, venous pooling.
2. **Neurogenic:** primary ANS failure (Shy Drager), secondary failure (stroke).

Vasovagal syncope: Faintness or loss of consciousness due to reflex reduction in blood pressure, precipitated by fear, anxiety or due to situational (urination, coughing or large meal). No loss of bladder, bowl function, or consciousness.

(Z): Shy-Drager: (Multiple System Atrophy with postural hypotension) ANS failure: orthostatic hypotension, olivopontocerebellar atrophy affecting balance, abnormal bladder and bowel control, impotence, gastroparesis & Parkinson disease (striatonigral degeneration). Death occurs within 7 to 10 years as a result of pneumonia or cardiopulmonary arrest.
Rx: L-dopa, dietary increases of salt and fluid & alpha-adrenergic medications.

Subclavian Steal Syndrome: The occlusion of left subclavian artery proximal or innominate artery causes symptoms of vertebrobasilar insufficiency that worsens when metabolic demand increases or with exercise of the affected arm. This causes motor difficulties, vertigo, syncope, & visual deficits (diplopia) due to diverted blood flow from the brain resulting in ischemia in the posterior cerebral circulation. The brachial systolic blood pressure of affected arm is >20 mmHg than normal arm.

Check: Arterial circulation with ultrasound or MRA.

CN IX: Glossopharyngeal nerve exits the brain through the jugular foramen. Function includes posterior 1/3 taste, swallowing, movement of the palate, afferent limb of gag reflex, salivation (parotid gland), monitoring carotid body, & sinus.

Check: uvula, soft palate, & gag reflex.

CN IX lesion: Peripheral Neuropathy: infection (*Corynebacterium Diphtheria*).

Glossopharyngeal Neuralgia: Stabbing pain in root of tongue.

Macroglossia: ddx Amyloidosis, neoplasm, or vascular hamartoma.

CN IX & CN X: Gag reflex (LMN), hyperactive gag reflex (UMN), & dysphagia (nucleus ambiguus).

CN X: Vagus nerve exits the brain through the jugular foramen: taste, swallowing, palate elevation, efferent limb of gag reflex, & parasympathetic function to most abdominal organs.

Test by asking patient to say "Kuh-Kuh" (checks palate elevation). Ask patient to say "E" (tests recurrent laryngeal nerve). Observe if uvula deviates. If the uvula does deviates away from the side of the lesion, then suspect medullary abnormality, Pancoast tumor.

S/s: hoarseness, dysphagia, loss of cough, & gag reflex.

Carotid sinus reflex: Pressure on carotid sinus slows heart rate.

Hypersensitive carotid sinus reflex: Syncope.

Oculocardiac reflex: Pressure of eye causes a decrease in heart rate via the afferent V1 to efferent CN X.

Recurrent laryngeal palsy ddx: left: Aortic aneurysm, thyroid surgery, & malignancy.

CN XI: Accessory nerve passes the jugular foramen (sternocleidomastoid & trapezius)
Test: ask patient to move head to side & shrug shoulders.

CN XI LESIONS: If lesion exists, then head deviates away from lesion.

CN XII: Hypoglossal nerve passes through hypoglossal canal.
Check: for tongue movements (fasciculations), midline protrusion & atrophy of tongue. Ask patient to make following sounds "La la, tee tee & dee dee" (check tongue movement).

CN XII LESIONS: *LMN* lesion deviates *toward* the lesion when tongue is protruded. *UMN lesion* - tongue *deviates* to the opposite side.

SUMMARY OF MOTOR & SENSORY CN
MOTOR CN: III, IV, VI, XI & XII.
SENSORY CN: I, II & VIII.
MIX CN: V, VII, IX & X.

MULTIPLE CN ABNORMALITIES

Cavernous sinus lesion: Symptoms include vision change, headache, neurologic manifestations of lesions to CN III, IV, V_1 & VI. Classic symptoms: look for *head or neck infection with venous obstruction and opthalmoplegia.*
Risk factors: malignancy, DM, mucormycosis, upper respiratory organisms, & immunosuppressed patients.
Check: CBC, ESR, blood cultures, MRI with contrast is diagnostic test of choice. Diagnosis has poor prognosis.
Rx: ICU, IV fluids, antibiotics, and supportive care.

Cerebellopontine angle lesion: Symptoms associated with V, VII and/or VIII abnormalities and/or ataxia. (Acoustic neuroma), cerebello-pontine angle
Rx: shrink tumor (Gamma knife or radiation) & surgery.

(Z): Foster Kennedy: Meningioma: Ipsalateral: Olfactory + Optic atrophy & gradual unilateral symptoms.

(Z): Jugular Foramen Syndrome: Unilateral IX- XI
ddx: glomus tumor nasopharyngeal cancer & aneurysms.

(Z): Sarcoidosis: usually female in the 20-40 years old, CN lesions to II- IV & VI-VII. Definitive diagnosis made by histology; classic chest imaging findings reveals bilateral hilar adenopathy during stage II & III of disease; biopsy significant for "non-caseating granulomas." Other lesions include uveitis, cataracts, blindness, seizures, & peripheral neuropathy. Only 5% of sarcoidosis is isolated to CNS.
Check: chest CAT scan, calcium levels, ACE levels (may be

elevated) & perform an ophthalmologic exam. Galium scan helpful.

Rx: corticosteroids.

SENSORY EXAMINATION TECHNIQUES

Test: Pin prick, thermal sensation (usually with cold object), deep pain in the comatose, light touch, vibration (with 128 hz tuning fork), & position (proprioception).
Check: graphesthesia, paresthesia, stereognosis, simultaneous stimulation.

Graphesthesia: Trace figure identification. Have patient close eyes then draw a test number in their extended hand. After the test number (tell them which number it is as it is being drawn), draw a number (large size) in the hand and ask for identification. Repeat 3 times then switch hands. Provide test number for both hands. Failure is less than 2/3 numbers.

Paresthesia: Tingling, pins & needles sensation.

Dysesthesias: Unpleasant abnormal sensation experienced suddenly without stimulation, commonly seen in Diabetics.

Stereognosis: Object identification.

Simultaneous stimulation (extinction)**:** If perceives on one side, it is indicative of parietal lobe lesion.

(Z): Arsenic poisoning: Painful sensation, throat constriction, dysphagia.
Check: for Mees lines seen in chronic disease (horizontal white bands of the nails) & blood levels.

Rx: removal from exposure, **Dimercaprol**, **Penicillamine**, gastric lavage, & hemodialysis (HD).

Cauda Equina Syndrome: Caused by disk herniation or tumor commonly. L3–S5 roots, manifested by gradual & unilateral severe radicular pain in a dermatomal distributions especially in the leg, muscle wasting asymmetric & unilateral sensory loss, unilateral saddle shape paresthesia; poor anal sphincter tone, often bladder & bowel sphincter function is affected late in the disease, ankle & knee jerks may be absent.
Check: CT scan with & without contrast or lumbar myelogram, or MRI, EMG/nerve conduction study.
Rx: neurosurgical emergency: decompression of the spinal canal via laminectomy within 48 hours of the onset of symptoms making recovery possible.

Conus medullaris syndrome: Causes include lumbar stenosis, spinal trauma (most injuries of T11 & L2); symptoms include sudden pain, bilateral saddle shape sensory distribution, sensory dissociation, fasciculations, normal knee reflex, ankle jerk affected, back pain, & decrease sexual function (impotence).
Check: CT scan, MRI with contrast.
Rx: emergency decompression of the spinal canal via laminectomy within 48 hours of the onset of symptoms.

Diabetic Neuropathy: Peripheral neuropathy symmetric "stocking-glove" sensory loss numbness, burning, femoral neuropathy, 3rd CN palsy, Charcot's joints (destruction of weight bearing weight joints); EMG: denervation.
Rx: foot care, pain control: Gabapentin, Oxcarbazine, Carbamazepine, & Amitriptyline.

ddx of Stocking-glove sensory loss: DM, thyroid disease, uremia, dysproteinemia (multiple myeloma), HIV, amyloidosis, vitamin B-12 deficiency, iatrogenic (chemotherapy, chronic steroid use), alcohol abuse, heavy metal intoxication, lupus, cervical cord lesion, & lyme disease.

ddx of transient incontinence (DIAPPERS IS): **D**elirium/ confused state, **I**nfection (urinary/URI), **A**trophic (urethritis, vaginitis) **P**harmaceuticals (diuretics), **P**sychological (excess H_2O intake), **E**xcessive urine output (diabetes mellitus, CHF), **R**estricted mobility, **S**tool impaction, **I**diopathic (Normal pressure hydrocephalus), & **S**ensory deficit.
Check: post-void residual urine volume, urinalysis, & most important detailed history/physical exam.

Drug induced incontinence: Antihistamines, antidepressants (tricyclic), antiadrenergics (clonidine), anticholinergics, antipsychotics, β blockers, α blockers, calcium channel blockers, ACE inhibitor, ETOH, & diuretics.

Overflow incontinence: Urine retained in the bladder causes the bladder to reach maximum capacity. The bladder then leaks urine due to "overflow." The bladder is underactive due to medications, obstruction of urine outflow due to prostate or denervation due to diabetes (neurogenic incontinence). Patients tend to dribble & have decreased force of urine stream.
Rx: intermittent catheterization, indwelling or suprapubic catheterization.

Stress incontinence: Malfunction of urethral sphincter due to pelvic prolapse or displacement of the urethra & bladder neck that causes urine to escape when intra-abdominal pressure increases (laughter).

This causes the bladder pressure to be greater than the urethral pressure resulting in urine loss. Other causes include congenital, surgical damage to intrinsic sphincter.

Rx: **Kegel exercises**, bladder training, α-adrenergic medications, estrogen, pessary (for patients with uterine prolapse).

Urge incontinence "overactive bladder": Uncontrolled bladder contractions that can not be inhibited by cerebral centers. The contractions are due to inflammation or irritation within the bladder.

Rx: behavioral therapies (bladder training, Kegel exercises), then Oxybutynin (SE: dry mouth). If all else fails, consider surgery. **Other medications: Tolterodine:** similar to **Oxybutynin, Propantheline:** anticholinergic agent**, Dicyclomine:** antispasmodic**.**

Intervertebral disc herniation: Acute lancinating pain, common C6-C7 then C6-C7 & L5, S1. The nucleus pulposus herniates due to an annulus fibrosis defect, usually in the posterolateral area, which is the weakest point.

Check: x-ray, spinal MRI, CT myelogram, EMG & NCS.

Rx: **NSAIDS,** muscle relaxants, physical therapy & surgery.

If herniation at:
- **C5:** Symptoms from herniation of C4-C5 will cause sensory deficit of upper lateral arm & elbow. Motor deficit includes deltoid muscle weakness.
- **C6:** Symptoms from herniation of C5-C6 will cause sensory deficit of lateral forearm, thumb, and index finger. Motor deficit includes biceps and extensor carpi radialis longus/brevis weakness & deltoid muscle.
- **L4:** Symptoms from herniation of L3-L4 will cause decrease

patellar tendon reflex with sensory deficit in the posterolateral thigh, anterior knee and medial leg. Motor deficit of knee & foot extension is observed.

- **L5:** Symptoms from herniation of L4-L5 then decreased sensation over lateral calf, anterior lateral leg, dorsum of the foot & great toe. Motor deficit of the extensor hallucis longus & brevis is observed.
- **S1**: Decreased ankle reflex, decreased sensation of lateral malleolus, & lateral foot. Motor deficit includes peroneus longus & brevis, gastrocnemius-soleus complex.

Important to note that lumbar discs usually compress the nerve root exiting one interspace below it. **Neglect:** Lack of attention or unresponsive to stimulus on opposite side of nondominant parietal lobe. (see brain section)

Radiculopathy: Sharp pain, asymmetric, weakness atrophy, fasciculation, & sensory loss. Neurologic emergency needs treatment in less than 24hrs.

Spurling test: Evaluates cervical nerve root impingement. The patient extends neck & rotates then laterally bends head to symptomatic side. Pressure is applied to patient's head. Test is positive if radicular arm pain results in the distribution of spinal nerve.

Meningeal Neurosyphilis: Tabetic Neurosyphilis: Type of neurosyphilis: posterior roots of the spinal cord, resulting in ataxia, hypotonia, impotence, constipation, hypotonic bladder, areflexia, general paresis, & Romberg sign (+). Other findings include Argyll Robertson pupils, optic atrophy, & Charcot joints (decrease sensation of lower extremities) in most patients.
Check: serum: fluorescent treponemal antibody-absorption test +

CSF: lymphocytic pleocytosis, oligoclonal bands& VDRL positive.
Rx: IV **aqueous procaine penicillin G** 2-4 million units IM. If allergic to penicillin use: 1) Tetracycline 2) Erythromycin.

(Z): Jarisch-Herxheimer reaction: Inflammation signs & symptoms of fever, chills, new rash after antibiotic administered. The antibiotic causes the spirochete to breakdown and releases its endotoxin.
Rx: antipyretics & antihistamine.

(Z): Westphal's sign: Loss of knee jerk (Tabes dorsalis).

Meralgia Paresthesia: Compression of lateral femoral cutaneous nerve originating from L2 and L3 causes burning numbness sensation of lateral thigh that worsens when patient walks down stairs or remains standing for long periods. The symptoms may be reproduced by palpation of inguinal ligament (anterior superior iliac spine). The condition is benign and occurs in last trimester of pregnancy, obese patients, truckers, or in trauma patients.
Rx: weight loss & steroids.

(Z): Mercury Poison: Sensory neuropathy (paresthesia)

Restless Leg Syndrome: Unpleasant limb sensation legs > arms, worsens with rest or evening/night, brief relief with movement. Primary causes include idiopathic CNS disorders. Secondary causes include iron deficiency anemia, folate, & magnesium deficiency.
Check: calcium, potassium, magnisum, ferritin.
Rx: pramipexole, ropinirole levodopa/carbidopa, pergolide, clonidine, & gabapentin. Stop antidepressants, calcium channel blockers, & caffeine.

Shingles (Herpes Zoster) & Postherpetic Neuralgia: Patients complain of a prodrome of burning pain, paresthesias or pruritus typically precedes the maculopapular rash that then evolves into a vesicle by 1 or 2 days. The virus enters the sensory dorsal root ganglia & follows a dermatomal distribution, commonly T5 & T6 described as a "belt-like pattern." The dermatomal distributions in order from most frequent to least: thoracic, trigeminal, cervical, lumbar, & sacral.

Rx: antiviral agents **Acyclovir** (Zovirax) within 72 hours of onset of rash.

Post-Herpetic neuralgia Rx: Generally a self-limited condition but can last indefinitely.

1. **Capsaicin.**
2. **Tricyclic Antidepressants:** Amitriptyline (Elavil), nortriptyline (Pamelor), imipramine (Tofranil)**,**
3. **Anticonvulsants:** Phenytoin (Dilantin), carbamazepine (Tegretol) and gabapentin (Neurontin). Famcyclovir has been shown to have decrease incidence of postherpetic neuralgia.

Syringomyelia: Central cavitation of the spinal cord of undetermined cause in a "cape distribution" of selective **p**ain/**t**emperature loss (spinothalamic), especially affects the intrinsic muscles of the hands. Patients have intact proprioception but LMN weakness (flaccid paralysis, atrophy that results from destruction of central spinal gray matter 2nd to trauma, associated with Arnold Chiari). **Check:** MRI & Myelogram.

Rx: surgical decompression & shunting of the cavity.

Spinal stenosis: Pain worsens as day progresses, but is relieved by rest, +/- bladder/bowl dysfunction MRI, CT +/- myelograph.

Rx: laminectomy.

Thalamic Pain Syndrome: (syndrome of Déjérine Roussy): Spontaneous excruciating pain on side opposite of vascular lesion (ventral posterior lateral VPL/ ventral posterior medial nuclei VPM), mild hemiplegia, & sensory disturbance including astereognosis (inability to identify objects in the hand). Commonly due to small stroke (lacunar infarction) localized to the thalamus.

MOTOR DEFINITIONS

Important to Check for tone, and strength.

Grade = indication.
0 = no muscle movement observed
    1 = trace visible movement but no movement at the joint
    2 = movement at the joint, but not against gravity
    3 = movement against gravity but not against added resistance
    4= movement against resistance but not normal strength
    5= normal strength

Asterixis: Hands jerk after being provoked by having patient extend arms, dorsiflex wrists, & spread the fingers; tremor-like seen in hepatic/metabolic encephalopathy.

Athetosis: Involuntary irregular, slow muscle contractions in hands (fingers) may indicate basal ganglia lesion, Cerebral palsy, Lesch-Nyhan syndrome or Kernicterus.

Chorea: Rapid, irregular unpredictable, brief jerks from one part of body to other random sequence. Purposeless movement; patient cannot keep tongue out; inability to keep tight hand grip.

ddx chorea: Drug induced (cocaine, L-dopa), cerebral infarction (Basal ganglia), inflammation (SLE, Chorea Gravidarum), Neurodegenerative (Huntington chorea), infectious (poststreptococcal Sydenham Chorea), hyperthyroid, carbon monoxide poisoning, & pregnancy.

Dystonia: Co-contraction of agonist/antagonist muscles, slow sustained movement. Causes include basal ganglion lesion, metabolic disorders, degenerative disorders, or side effect of medications, i.e. neuroleptics. The condition can worsen from fatigue & stress.

Fasciculations: Spontaneous contraction of *all* of the muscle fibers belonging to a single motor unit that does not cause movement at a joint, coarser form of muscular contraction than fibrillation. They occur as a result of peripheral neuropathy, dehydration, or fatigue.

Fibrillation: Spontaneous contractions of *individual* muscle fiber due to denervation.

Flaccid: Absence of tone, no muscle resistance.

Hemiballism: Spontaneous, ballistic, flailing, irregular arm/leg movements on one side of body. Lesion at the caudate nucleus & subthalamic nucleus as a result of a stroke should be suspected. **Rx:** Reserpine, Haloperidol, or ventrolateral thalamotomy.

Muscle disease: Wasting usually proximal muscles with decrease tone.

Myoclonus: Spontaneous, rapid brief twitching of a group of muscles that move a limb across a joint.

ddx: metabolic, urea-cycle defects, hyperthyroid, degenerative disorders, prion disease (Creutzfeldt-Jakob) & trauma.

Spastic: Increase muscle tension with passive stretch, resistance increases with increase velocity; "clasp knife" indicative of corticospinal tract lesion.

Tandem walking: heel to toe. Check midline cerebellar functions. Other tests for midline cerebellar function include Heel-shin test.

MOTOR DISEASES

ALS: Amyotrophic **L**ateral **S**clerosis (Lou Gehrig disease) M=F 40 years of age, classically both UMN & LMN
S/s:
1. UMN: spasticity, *hyperreflexia*, (Hoffman, Babinski, clonus) positive.
2. LMN: distal muscle *weakness/atrophy*, legs, hands, slurred speech, foot drop, decrease DTR, dysphagia & atrophic fasciculating tongue.
3. No sensory loss; does not affect bowls or bladder function.
   Check: EMG study (denervation) & nerve conduction velocities are normal, defective gene that codes for superoxide dismutase on chromosome 21 & defective gene that code for neurofilament. Bad prognosis: death within 5 years of onset of disease usually due to respiratory failure.
   Rx: Riluzole (Rilutek): anti-glutamatergic medication that slows progression of disease
   Check LFT. SE: hepatotoxicity, asthenia (weakness), vertigo & paresthesia.
   For symptoms of spasticity use:
       1) Baclofen **2)** Valium **3)** Dantrolene.

For Pain:
1) NSAIDS 2) Anticonvulsants.

ddx of ALS: Spinal cord lesions (Syringomyelia), spinal bone lesions (metastatic tumors), infection (HIV), endocrine (DM), toxins (lead).

Cerebral palsy: History: cerebral anoxia at birth or prematurity. The cause is often multifactorial. Motor disturbances include spastic diplegia, spastic hemiplegia, spastic quadriplegia, & (dyskinetic) choreoathetosis & ataxia.

Huntington Chorea: Ages 35-40, gradual behavior changes, progression to chorea, dementia, & psychosis. MRI (cerebral/caudate nucleus atrophy, CAG repeats (Cytosine, Adenine & Guanine) which codes for glutamine, genetic anticipation. This causes disease to manifest at earlier age found on chromosome 4p, autosomal dominant.
Rx: **Haldol** (for chorea). Xenazine (tetrabenazine) (for chorea).

Hemiballismus: Random violent unilateral flailing limbs as a result of damage to the subthalamic nucleus (glutamatergic neurons) causes include stroke, tumor, or infectious process.

Parkinson's: Resting tremor (3-4 Hz), "pin rolling" bradykinesia, postural instability, festinating gait (shuffling gait), cogwheel rigidity, masked like facies, micrography & (retro)pulsion, postural reflex impairment (responses that control the position of the trunk & extremities as a result falls; gait or balance problems).
Pathology: Dopa levels decrease in basal ganglia with degeneration of neural tracts of Substantia Nigra. Lewy bodies (intracytoplasmic

inclusions) cause Uni to Bi resting tremor that discontinues with sleep or movement. DTR are normal.

Rx:

1. **Benztropine mesylate** (Cogentin) anticholinergic (do not use if patient has BPH, angle-closure glaucoma, GI obstruction) SE: paralytic ileus, urinary retention & hyperthermia.
   Other anticholinergics:
   - **Biperiden** (Akineton) SE: tachycardia, dry mouth, blurry vision & delirium.
   - **Trihexyphenidyl** (Artane) controls extrapyramidal disorders caused by CNS medications. SE: similar to Biperiden.

2. **Sinemet:** carbidopa/dopa
   Side effect: Dyskinesias, on/off phenomena: the patient will have hypokinesia/hyperkinesia periods as the effectiveness of levodopa therapy comes and goes, seemingly unrelated to dose times & NMS.

3. **Dopamine agents:** Amantadine, Atamet, Bromocriptine (Parlodel), Levodopa, Pergolide (Permax), Pramipexole (Mirapex), Ropinirole (Requip), Selegiline, & Sinemet.

   3a. Amantadine (Symmetrel): endogenous dopamine release from presynaptic clefts. SE: difficult urination especially in elderly.

   3b. (Z): Bromocriptine (dopamine agonist): old drug not used in the US, but tested on boards; SE: confusion; hallucinations (seeing, hearing); uncontrolled movements of the body, face, tongue, arms, hands & head.

   3c. Selegiline (Eldepryl: decrease dopamine reuptake) MAO-B inhibitor. (See side effect section)

   3d. Levodopa: SE: dyskinesia, motor fluctuations, vivid dreams, nightmares & psychosis.

4. **COMT inhibitors: Entacapone** (Comtan) & **Tolcapone** (Tasmar) enhance the effect of levodopa/carbidopa, the medications help with improving muscle control.
   SE: Black box warning: acute fulminant liver failure, neuroleptic malignant syndrome & confusion.

5. **Surgery:**

   1. (Palliative vs. restorative) Globus Pallidus internal-segment pallidotomy (relieve the dyskinesias seen with levodopa therapy)

   2. Deep brain stimulation (effective for tremor and for relieving dyskinesias)

   3. Restorative surgery use of fetal nigral transplantation (controversial & controversial) or gene therapy.

Cogwheel rigidity: Lead pipe & extrapyramidal lesion.

Festinating gait: Narrow based shuffling gait, patients try to catch up with their center of gravity in Parkinson's.

Atypical Parkinson: "Parkinson-plus syndromes" no tremor, symmetric, unstable blood pressure & progress more rapidly. The patients lose their dopamine receptor function as a result. These patients do not respond to levodopa.

Drug induced Parkinson: Don't give this to your Parkinson patients! Haloperidol, prochlorperazine, reserpine, tetrabenazine, MPTP, Metoclopramide, phenothiazine (blocks dopa), CO & magnesium poison.

"Parkinson-plus syndromes" (multisystem degeneration): Shy Drager, progressive supranuclear palsy, multiple system atrophy, & Parkinsonism-Dementia complex.

TREMORS

Benign essential tremor: (familial tremor) Autosomal dominant (AD) in 50% of cases, action tremor especially hands, but can also affect head, voice, and legs. Low frequency tremor of 4-12 Hz. Improves with ETOH & worsens with nicotine, caffeine, anxiety, stress, fatigue & cold temperatures.
Rx:
1. **Propranolol** SE: bradycardia.
2. **Primidone** SE: urinary retention & depression.
3. **Benzodiazepines.**

Cerebellar tremor: Low frequency (< 5 Hz) caused by lesions of the lateral cerebellar nuclei or superior cerebellar peduncle, or its connections, causes intention tremor (multiple sclerosis, trauma, tumors, strokes and hereditary ataxias).
Check: gait, rapid & alternating movements.

Resting tremor: Basal ganglion lesion seen in Parkinson disease (see Parkinson disease), ETOH withdrawal, neurosyphillis.

Tremor ddx: Physiologic tremor, drug induced: lithium OD, haloperidol, metoclopramide, β-agonist, valproate sodium & alcohol withdrawal.

Myelopathy: Triad of clinical findings:

1. Bilateral UMN weakness of the legs or arms (paraparesis, paraplegia)

2. Bilateral impairment of sensation with a "level" that separates normal sensation from a region of impaired sensation.

3. Bowel or bladder sphincter dysfunction

Poliomyelitis 3 serotypes (P1, P2 & P3): Young age, headache, fever, stiff neck, muscle pain, asymmetric paralysis LMN, & no sensory component. No superficial reflexes. CSF: increase protein/WBC, lymphocytic pleocytosis. Transmitted via fecal-oral, Salk (killed inactivated poliovirus vaccine [IPV]) administered subcutaneus; Sabin vaccine is an oral attenuated live poliovirus vaccine that can cause polio. The USA only uses the IPV form of the vaccine. **Dx:** isolation of throat, feces, & increase in polio antibody titers.

Transverse Myelitis: Occurs in adults & children ages 10-19 & 30-39 demyelinating disorder of the spinal cord. The inflammatory process localized over both sides of one level or segments of the spinal cord; abrupt onset of weakness to the arms, legs; Sensory disturbance includes back pain, paresthesias in the legs, trunk with proprioception & vibration spared. Other symptoms include loss of bowel control with urinary retention. Disease occurs as a result of post vaccination & post infectious. 1/3 will fully recover with the ability to walk but will have minimal bowel, bladder and paresthesias. 1/3 will have fair recovery but will have significant spastic gait, sensory dysfunction, and incontinence. The last 1/3 will have no recovery and remain wheelchair or bedridden. **Labs: CSF: pleocytosis with increase protein, normal glucose, MRI or myelography (rule out compression of spinal cord). Rx:** Supportive, IV methylprednisolone for demyelinating or post infections causes suspected.

Tics: Abrupt, repetitive movements at irregular intervals.
ddx: idiopathic, stroke, & drug induced.

Tourette Syndrome: Male, usually seen before age of 18 years old; patients may have history of OCD, ADHD, learning disorder, conduct disorder, oppositional defiant disorder. Symptoms include multiple motor repetitions manifesting themselves by vocal tics (grunting, shouting), coprolalia (obscenities) or movements of the extremities. The symptoms are present for more than 1 year in order to make the diagnosis.
Rx: Fluphenazine, Haldol or **Pimozide** are helpful with tics. **Clonidine & SSRI** help with behavior symptoms.

(Z): Tic bite paralysis:
S/s: muscle pain & paraesthesia, ascending flaccid paralysis, absent DTR, anorexia, lethargy, muscle weakness, incoordination, nystagmus (toxin-secreting *Ixodes*), & normal CSF.
Rx: removal of tic.

Pediatric (Z): Werdnig-Hoffman (spinal muscular atrophy I):
Failure in development of anterior horn cells causes paresis of limb muscles, no DTR, with onset at/shortly after birth. Death occurs in 1-2 years as a result of respiratory failure.
Note: Polio also affects anterior horn but usually seen later in life. This disease is autosomal recessive and autosomal dominant.

SPINAL TRACTS

Corticobulbar tract: Descending pathway from cerebral cortex to internal capsule to (1st order) nucleus 7th CN to (2nd order) tomuscles of facial expression. Upper face: bilateral innervations from UMN. Lower face: contralateral input from LMN. The fibers of this pathway terminate in the brain stem where the motor nuclei of CN V, VII, IX, X, XI, & XII & optomotor nuclei of CN III, IV, & VI are located.

Corticospinal: Cerebral cortex to medullary pyramid decussates then continues as lateral corticospinal tract.
Voluntary muscle **Test**: arms out with eyes closed (pronator drift), spread finger against resistance, rapid tapping movement, DTR reflexes, Hoffman reflex, & Babinski.

Dorsal column: Tactile discriminations, vibration, & proprioception. Encapsulated nerve ending to dorsal column to nucleus & Gracilis fasciculus + Cuneate fasciculus to cross-internal arcuate, fiber of medulla to ascend in the medial lemniscus to nucleus VPL of the thalamus to 1°, 2° sensory cortex.

a. Gracile fasciculus: ipsilateral loss of tactile, position, & vibration of leg; "Graceful dancer"
b. Cuneate fasciculus: ipsilateral loss of tactile, position, & vibration of arm.

S*P*ino*Th*alamic: *P*ain & *T*emperature one level below lesion, input via fast A type & slow C type. Fibers cross-anterior white commissure then anterolateral spinothalamic tract to nucleus ventralis posterior lateral (VPL) & nonspecific nuclei of thalamus to 1° + 2° sensory cortex.

LMN lesion: Damage to motor neurons, flaccid paralysis, hypotonia, atrophy, fasciculations, fibrillation, areflexia or decrease DTR, & weakness.

UMN lesion: Spastic paresis and pyramidal symptoms (Babinski), decrease muscle swinging while walking, increase clonus, & arm pronation.

Anterior spinal artery infarct: Vertebral fracture or a herniated intervertebral disk causes bilateral; loss of pain & temperature (one level below lesion), with paresis/flaccid paralysis at the level of infarct usually legs>arms. Spares posterior column (Position, proproception & vibration sense). Pt has poor prognosis.

Anterior cord syndrome: Flexion injury involves complete loss of motor function with loss of temperature sensation distal to the lesion, with preservation of vibration and proprioception. **Rx:** surgical management.

Brown-Séquard: Lateral hemisection of the spinal cord, proprioception loss & weakness (corticospinal) occur ipsilateral to the lesion, while pain & temperature loss (spinothalamic) occur contralateral one level below. This is caused from penetrating injury or tumor.

Central cord syndrome: Most common incomplete cervical lesion caused by hyperextension resulting in weakness greater in arms compared to legs with sacral sensory sparing.

DEMENTIA & DELIRIUM

DEMENTIA: DSM-IV, **A**cquired memory impairment and with at least one additional acquired cognitive deficit: **A**bstract thought, **A**mnesia, **A**phasia

Agnosia: Inability to recognize or comprehend the meaning of various items despite intact sensory function.

Apraxia: Difficulty in carrying out skilled or purposeful motor activities despite intact motor function, although the object can be named and its uses described.

Chronic & insidious presentation, rule out delirium.

ddx: Alzheimer, multi infarct, HIV/AIDS; not reversible (usually), normal arousal level. Can be seen with Parkinson's (advanced), Normal Pressure Hydrocephalus, Chronic Subdural Hematomas, Huntington's disease, Pick's disease, Wilson's disease, Down's Syndrome (over the age of 35) and many others diseases.
Check: TSH, RPR, CBC, metabolic panel, B12 Folate levels, ESR, & Mini-Mental State examination (MMSE) (< 25) includes orientation, attention, concentration, general knowledge, memory, abstract thinking & calculations. MMSE may yield false positive in depression. May consider EEG/LP if prior head injury, staring spells, changes on MRI, relatively young age, and fulminant onset of memory loss (sudden over less than one year).

Mini-Mental status Exam:
    Time: year, season, date, day, month (5 points)
    Place: state, county, town, hospital, floor (5 points)
    Objects: pen, bed, watch (3 points)
    Serial 7, or spell World backwards (5 pts)
    Ask for three obects to be repeated (3 pts)
    Naming "pencil" and "watch" (2 pts)
    Repeat No ifs and or buts (1 pts)
    3-stage: take pencil or paper in your right hand, fold it in half, and put it on the floor. (3 pts)
    Read and obey command "Close your eyes" (1pts)
    Write a sentence (1pts)
    Copy a design. (1)

AIDS dementia complex: Initial symptoms include cognitive impairment, confusion, lack of concentration, impaired motor performance. Patients will have cortical atrophy (behavior change) & PET: decrease cortex utilization.

Dx: (by exclusion of other causes) depression & metabolic and infection

Check: MRI & CT to rule out other causes.

Rx: respond to antiretroviral therapy.

Alzheimer's: Spacial disorientation & impaired recent memory (temporal/parietal lobe) "will misplace things," but long-term memory is preserved. Patients will have impaired judgment, impaired intellect, shallow labile affect, loss of initiation & impaired abstract thinking.

Remember this is a "diagnosis by exclusion."

Risk factors include Down syndrome (21), female, family history & age. Definitive diagnosis made by autopsy. Common pathological findings include Hirano Bodies Neurofibrillary Tangles, mutations: in apolipoprotein E-4 on chromosome 19, amyloid precursor gene at 21q21, genes coding for presenilin-1, presenilin-2 on chromosome 14 & 1 respectively.

Check: mini mental status exam (refer to section on dementia for work up), Complications: "Sun-downing" & falls.

Rx:

1. Cholinesterase inhibitors: **Tacrine**: SE: liver toxicity, nausea, vomit, seizures, syncope (Now rarely prescribed.).

2. **Donepezil** (Aricept): SE: hepatic, insomnia, cholinergic manifestations: diarrhea, salivation.

3. **Rivastigmine** (Exelon): SE: asthenia, respiratory depression, urinary obstruction & seizures.

4. **Galantamine** (Reminyl): SE: seizures, syncope & hypotension

5. **Memantine (Namenda): SE**: confusion, dizziness.

Prevention Rx (suggested): Estrogen replacement in post menapausal women, NSAIDS, Vitamin E, Statins & Screening for sleep apnea.

(Z): Gerstmann-Straüssler: Hereditary autosomal dominant symptoms include ataxia, myoclonus & slowly progressive dementia. Spongiform encephalopathy (vacuolation within nerve and glial cells).

Lewy Body Dementia: Combination of dementia & Parkinsons with extrapyramidal symptoms, recurrent visual hallucinations, fluctuating cognition, and spontaneous motor features of Parkinsonism. Other supportive of diagnosis symptoms include falls, syncope & systematized delusions.
Male > female 2:1, average time from onset to death is 6.4 years with cause of death being aspiration pneumonia.
Rx: Donepezil & dopamine agonist. Avoid antipsychotics may exacerbate Parkinsons disease.

Pseudobulbar Palsy: Inappropriate emotional outbursts, dysarthria, swallowing difficulties & ↑ DTR.

Picks: Female 60 y/o, progressive dementia, predominate frontal (personalitychanges), temporal lobe (behavior/speech changes, precede memory changes), loss of personal awareness, pick bodies: basophilic cytoplasmic inclusions found in the cortex. MRI: atrophy of frontal & anterior temporal lobes.

Vascular Dementia (Multi-infarct Dementia): cortical strokes, increase risk factors include: male, smoking, hypertension, & "step-wise progression of disease" (pseudobulbar effect).

Symptoms include changes in gait, incontinence. CT: multiple infarcts to brain.

REVERSIBLE CAUSES OF DEMENTIA: Wernicke, Vitamin B-12 deficiency, normal pressure hydrocephalus, CNS infection, depression, medication side effects, dehydration, hypothyroid, hypoglycemia & hyponatremia.

Korsakoff Syndrome: Severe memory impairment & confabulations. This condition is irreversible. Patients are not able to process new information. It is important to give vitamin B1 (thiamine deficiency in alcoholics) before glucose; affects the bilateral mamillary bodies.

Normal Pressure Hydrocephalus (NPH): (classic triad)
1. Ataxia
2. Dementia
3. Urinary incontinence: etiology includes infection, idiopathic, neoplasm. Pt will not have headache. In the elderly, LP is diagnostic & therapeutic.

Check: CT & MRI (enlarge ventricles), isotope cisternography.
Rx:
1. V-A or V-P shunt complications of shunts: E. coli, Staphylococcal Aureus & Staphylococcal Epidermidis.
2. **Acetazolamide** SE: metabolic acidosis, altered taste & tinnitus. No definitive evidence exists that shows medication to be successful treatment for NPH.

Pseudodementia: Mimics dementia but cause is not due to brain dysfunction but due to depression. The new terminology is "dementia of depression."

Wernicke-Korsakoff: Ophthalmoplegia, nystagmus, gait abnormalities, confabulations, recent memory loss, irreversible. Atrophy of superior cerebellar tonsil; due to alcohol over-exposure. **Rx:** vitamin B1 (Thiamine) x 3 days.

Wernicke Encephalopathy: Acute onset, Ataxia, ophthalmoplegia (nystagmus, weakness or paralysis of external rectus muscle), & confusion (consciousness disturbances & drowsiness).

Delirium: "change in sensorium"
DSM-IV Criteria:

1. Acute onset symptoms develop over a short period of time

2. Fluctuating change in cognition (confused state, hallucinations & illusions) & disturbance of consciousness

ddx: 2nd to polypharmacy, infection, metabolic hypo (hyper)-natremia, renal failure, hypothyroid, nutritional & endocrine. **Rx:** underlying cause.

GAIT

Test Cerebellar:

Check Finger to nose, heel-knee-shin, tandem gait, dysdiadochokinesis & tap heels with ankles dorsiflexed.

(Z): Antalgic limp: Patient limits weight on limb 2nd to pain.

Ataxia: (inferior cerebellar peduncle or by dysfunction of the pathways leading into and out of the cerebellum.) Uncontrolled falling occurs.

Ataxic gait: Indicates cortical integration of movement is abnormal.

Cerebellar Ataxic: Veers to side of lesion, wide base gait
   ddx: phenytoin, ETOH, multiple sclerosis, & CVD.

Gradual Ataxia ddx: Vitamin E deficiency, hypothyroid & hereditary disorders.

Hemiplegic ddx: UMN: Stroke, & multiple sclerosis.

(Z): Marche Apatites Pas: Patient takes small steps; bilateral diffuse cortical dysfunction: CVA.

Sudden Ataxia ddx: Stroke, brain hemorrhage, & head trauma.

(Z): Scissoring: Indicates spastic paraparesis
   ddx: Cerebral palsy & cord compression.

(Z): Sensory Ataxia: Wide base gait, Romberg +, peripheral neuropathy, & posterior column loss; patient watches his steps.

(Z): Waddling: Weak, ineffective proximal muscles
   ddx: bilateral congenital hip dislocation, proximal myopathies, abdominal protrudes, lordosis is common.

HEADACHES

Headaches: If you suspect a tumor, obtain a MRI with contrast, especially if patient has focal neurologic signs. Other alarming signs include new onset headaches especially in older adults (>40 years of age), awakening headache, new headaches in the immunosuppressed.

Headache ddx: hypoxia, **h**ypoglycemia, **h**ypercalcemia, & **h**ypernatremia, **h**ypertension; +other causes include CO toxicity, TMJ, bruxism.

Cluster headache: Male 25-50 year old, quick onset, 1-3 brief episodes lasting 30 minutes- 3 hours of periorbital pain over 24 hour period for 4-8 wks, followed by a 6 month to 1-year pain free period. Recurrent, severe stabbing, burning, unilateral orbitotemporal headaches that occurs at same time of year, associated with ipsa-lateral: photophobia, redness of eye, lacrimation & rhinorrhea, +/- headache precipitated by ETOH or vasodilating medications. No prodrome. Abortive **Rx:** 100% **O2** or **Sumatriptan, indomethacin, & Cafergot.** Prophylaxis: **Verapamil, ergotamine, cyproheptadine, indomethacin** or **Methysergide** (see drug list).

Migraine: Female, unilateral or diffuse pain that begins as a throbbing pain then becomes a dull ache; ask about family history & photophobia. If Aura prodrome (scintillating, scotoma, ataxia, N/V, then it is called a Classic migraine. The new term is **migraine with aura**, if common migraine now called "migraine without aura"
Vague signs & symptoms > 4 hrs –72 hrs. Other symptoms include depression, hunger & thirst. Migraine defined by 2 attacks with aura or five attacks without aura. Avoid triggers: skipping meals, red wine, smoking, dehydration, caffeine & sleep deprivation.

Tension headache: Most common type of headache
S/s: chronic contraction of the scalp/ mastication muscles, bilateral constant non-throbbing bandlike, squeezing pain, worsens as day progresses, headaches >15 days/month x 6 months. Patients are

devoid of typical migraine complains (photophobia, nausea, etc.).
Rx: muscle relaxer, analgesic (aspirin, acetaminophen).
Prophylaxis: Tricyclic antidepressants (amitriptyline).

OTHER TYPES:

(Z): Atypical Migraines: headache with neurological manifestations, as a result of brain vessels spasms.

S/s: Facial pain, motor symptoms (hemiparesis),

Rx: Dihydroergotamine, headache diet.

(Z): Basilar Migraines: Female transient brainstem signs (vertigo, tinnitus, perioral numbness & diplopia

(Z): Ophthalmoplegic Migraine: Compression of CN 3 & mydriasis.

Thunder Clap Headache: Sudden onset of severe headache, rule out subarachnoid bleed, ddx aneurysm & initial migraine.

COMMON HEADACHE MEDICATIONS AND THEIR SIDE EFFECTS:

1. **Ergotamine** derivatives example: **Dihydroergotamine Mesylate** (Migranal): contraindicated in sepsis, impaired renal or hepatic function, & coronary artery disease.
   SE: black box warning: peripheral ischemia, vasospasm, MI, arrhythmias.
2. **Sumatriptan** (Imitrex): Do not use on patients with coronary artery disease, uncontrolled hypertension or on 5-HT1 agonists, caution use with patients with cardiac risk factors.
   SE: coronary spasm, numbness, & weakness.

(Z): Other triptan include:

    a. Almotriptan: fewer SE than sumatriptan.

    b. Naratriptan: slowest onset of action.

    c. Rizatriptan: fastest onset of action.

3. NSAIDS **Naproxen** (Side effect: GI bleed). Combinations: **Excedrin Migraine** contains: (acetaminophen, aspirin & caffeine)
SE: Hepatotoxicity & bleeding. **Indomethacin** SE: GI bleed.

4. **Methysergide** (Sansert): give drug holiday
SE: Black Box warning: fibrosis of pulmonary, cardiac valve, & retroperitoneum. Others symptoms: ataxia & myalgia.

5. **Midrin** (acetaminophen, dichloralphenazone, isometheptene mucate): SE: hepatotoxicity, RTN, dizziness.

6. other meds to consider: antiemetics especially Reglan.

Migraine Prophylaxis:

1. **Beta-blockers (Propranolol/Timolol)**
SE: lassitude & depression. Limited use secondary to depression, impotence & hypotension; contraindicated in asthma, & heart block patients.

2. **Amitriptyline/imipramine** (Elavil): SE: non-specific ECG changes & changes in AV conduction, sedation, weight gain, & urinary retention.

3. **Valproic acid** (Depakote) SE: see anticonvulsion section.

4. **Verapamil** (Calan): SE: headache, bradycardia & heart block.

5. **Cyproheptadine** helps with prophylaxis treatment of pediatric migraine SE: urinary retention, hemolytic anemia & weight gain.

Other Headaches: Brain tumor, Carbon monoxide poisoning, encephalitis, meningitis, & postcoital headache.

Pregnancy: Migraines generally improve with pregnancy progression.

Pseudotumor Cerebri: Benign intracranial hypertension secondary to changes of CSF flow. Patients are obese female of childbearing age. **S/s:** bilateral papilledema, headache, N/V, blurry vision & tinnitus. **Test:** CT/MRI negative (normal imagining), CSF: high opening pressure (250-400 mm Hg) with normal differential. "Diagnosis by exclusion" Causes include SLE, nalidixic acid, tetracycline, withdrawal of steroids, and high dose of vitamins (especially vitamin A)
Rx: diuretic (acetazolamide), weight loss, surgery (lumboperitoneal cerebral spinal fluid shunt). Complication: Blindness or optic atrophy.

ddx for high opening pressure on CSF & normal brain scan: Pseudotumor cerebri, acute polyneuritis, & respiratory failure.

Post lumbar puncture headache: Headache within 48 hrs. of procedure; improves with lying down and worsens with erect position; self- limiting condition usually occurs within 3 days. Risk factors: needle size, pregnant. If headache persists, then consider epidural blood patch, IV caffeine, NSAIDS, encourage increase oral caffeine intake.

Temporal Arteritis: Female elderly with temporal headache, hx of polymyalgia rheumatic; jaw claudication, decrease pulse or pulseless, tender nodular temporal artery. Increase ESR > 55 mm/ hr; increase C-reactive protein, BX: mononuclear cell infiltrates.

Rx: High dose steroids helps prevents blindness. If patient has elevated ESR, start steroids before definitive diagnosis is made.

Tolosa Hunt (cavernous sinus syndrome) inflammatory disorder: Ophthalmoplegia, headache, & loss of sensation over forehead.

INFECTION DISEASES

Campylobacter: Gram negative rods, sudden onset with malaise, myalgia, arthralgia, & headache, cramping abdominal pain, diarrhea; demyelinating sequela in ascending fashion (G. Barré).

CMV: Ds-DNA associated with Guillain-Barré syndrome, encephalitis, radiculopathy, & retinitis (leading cause of visual loss).
Exam: hemorrhagic necrosis of retina, poor prognosis.
Infant - transmission across placenta, contact with urine, Saliva, and breast milk
Adults transmission by sexual or blood transfusion
Immunocompromised patients – can lead to interstitial pneumonitis & adrenal insufficiency.
Rx: Ganciclovir.

CMV infants: Mental retardation, microcephaly, sensorineural hearing loss, chorioretinitis, & periventricular calcifications.

Coxsackie A & B:
A: herpangina, hand foot mouth disease, myositis, flaccid paralysis; can be rapid and fatal.
B: myocarditis, CNS, focal myositis. Transmission is by fecal-oral aerosolization.
A/B: involves meninges, anterior horn cell & paralysis.

Creutzfeldt-Jacob: Rapid progressive dementia, myoclonus & choreoathetotic (jerks). Transmitted by corneal, dura grafts, Graft vs Host disease from cadaver, transplant. Prion disease can cause spongiform encephalopathy, loss of neurons, gliosis, & swelling. **CSF**: "14-3-3 protein". EEG 1-2 Hz, death within 6-7 months.

Echovirus: Aseptic meningitis transmission is by fecal-oral route.

HIV encephalitis: Progressive dementia; + motor changes.

HTLV-1: Gradual onset of myelopathy LE, optic atrophy spastic paraparesis, brisk DTR, urinary incontinence, with travel to Japan, & Caribbean (sexual contact, IV drugs).

Leprosy: *Mycobacterium leprae,* Pale anesthetic macular/nodular; + erythema lesion; + sensory changes.
Tuberculoid type: develops at the same time & has same distribution of skin.
Lepromatous type: Leonine facies, more sensory loss > in skin coolest areas. Motor deficit: superficial nerves: ulnar, median & peroneal nerve. The diagnosis is by physical exam & skin smear/biopsy.
Rx:

1. **Dapsone** SE: blood dyscrasia, sulfone syndrome, motor deficit like ALS.
2. **Clofazimine** SE: splenic infarct, & brown-black skin pigmentation.
3. **Rifampin.**

Lyme disorder: Skin, neurologic (Bells CN 7), ♥ conduction blocks, Borrelia burgdorferi, spirochete transmitted by *Ixodes scapularis*, the deer tick.

S/s: skin lesion, erythema chronicum migrans, is usually preceded or accompanied by fever, malaise, fatigue, headache, stiff neck; neurologic aseptic meningitis, ♥, articular manifestations, & radiculopathies. IgM ELISA + in arthritis may occur weeks to months later.
Rx: Doxycycline, Ceftriaxone (especially if neurologic signs & symptoms).

Mumps: Typically seen in late winter & spring with 14-24 day incubation period.
S/s: parotitis, septic meningitis, orchitis & pancreatitis. Sterility is rare.
Check: amylase, lipase & serology; vaccine is an attenuated virus, usually given at 12-15th months then at 4 to 6 years of age.

Progressive multifocal leukoencephalopathy (PML): White matter only, polyomavirus called the JC virus, motor weakness, clumsiness, personality changes, dementia, ataxia, & visual changes. Commonly seen with HIV (CD 4 < 100), immunosuppressed hosts.
Test: CT: hypodense white-matter lesion in the parietooccipital area. MRI: multiple focal well-defined white matter lesions that do not enhance or have mass effect. CSF: PCR for JC virus is diagnostic. Associated with lymphoma/leukemia, most will die within a year.

Rabies: Enveloped single stranded RNA, bullet shaped Negri bodies on brain biopsy, virus transmitted by bats/dogs and travels in a retrograde flow axoplasmic manner.
S/s: encephalitis, violent muscle contractions, ↑ lacrimation, ↑ salivation & hydrophobia. Other symptoms include incoordination, paresis & paralysis. Death is commonly due to

respiratory failure. Important to access the risk: If unprovoked animal attack, then considered high risk; important to capture animal and test for rabies. Animals with high risk include bats, skunks, non-domestic animals.

Rx: clean bite wound, +/- tetanus, immune globulin, vaccine. Rabies can be 100% fatal once symptoms develop.

(Z): Schistosoma Mansoni: Subacute paresis damage to **s**pinal cord. Patients tend to be **S**wimmers.

Rx: Praziquantel SE: dizziness, drowsiness & abdominal pain.

(Z): Subacute Sclerosing Panencephalitis: Caused by the **measles** virus, infection before 2 years old, followed by asymptomatic years, then gradual development of disease.

Check: EEG (periodic bursts), brain biopsy, CSF: oligoclonal IgG, elevated gamma globulin & anti-measles antibodies.

Stage I: progressive personality change, seizures

Stage II: Motor: myoclonus, ataxia, photosensitivity, ocular abnormalities & spasticity

Stage III: (Autonomic nervous system): Coma. Death usually occurs within 1-3 years.

Toxoplasmosis *gondii*: Cats, transplacental transmission, #1 CNS lesion with HIV, multiple ring enhancing lesions, large intracerebral cyst, typically in the basal ganglia. Diagnosis is by presence of antibody to toxoplasmosis. Bactrim prophylaxis if CD4 < 200. If patient does not improve with adequate treatment, it is important to rule out CNS lymphoma.

Rx:

1. **Pyrimethamine**: folate deficiency, hypersensitivity, blood dyscrasias.

2. **Sulfadiazine**: Steven Johnson's, Toxic Epidermal Necrolysis & crystalluria.

3. **Leucovorin** used to reduce folic acid toxicity.

MENINGITIS/TREATMENT

Meningitis: Photophobia & nuchal rigidity, fever, headache, nausea, changes in mental status, visual changes, ataxia, papilledema. **Early S/s**: lack of venous pulsations on retinal exam. Infants do not present with classic symptoms but rather are lethargic, irritable, poor feeding & hypo or (hyper)-thermia.

Brudzinski: Involuntary flexion of the knees & hips following flexion of the neck (*b*rain) indicates possible meningitis.

Leptomeninges: Arachnoid & pia most coomon site for meningitis.

Kernig sign patient is supine & the thigh is flexed at the trunk 90 degrees, complete extension of the leg (*K*ick) brings on pain; possible meningitis.

Risk factors: Parameningeal infections (mastoiditis, sinusitis), history of head trauma (fractures), anatomic defects (meningomyelocele), & immunosuppressed state.

Most specific test for evaluation of meningitis is csf culture. **Most sensitive**: csf Protein. **Best initial test**: Csf cell count.

Order CT before LP if: Focal findings, papilledema, altered mental status.

Rx: Ceftriaxone (treat before lumbar puncture).

Bacterial meningitis CSF: Decrease glucose, increase protein, increase PMN.

Viral meningitis CSF: NL glucose, increase protein, large increases in lymphocytes.

Fungal/TB: Decrease glucose, increase protein, lymphocytes increase. * very low levels of Glucose: meningoencephalitis due to lymphocytic choriomeningitis, Mumps or enterovirus.

Normal CSF values: Protein: 10-45 mg/dL, Glc: 48-80 mg/dL, Pressure: 60-180 mm H2O, Cell count: 0-5/HPF, CSF production in a day 400 - 500 cc/ 24 hrs (25 cc/hr).

Causes:

Adults:
1. Streptococcal pneumonia
2. Neisseria meningitis

Children meningitis:
1. Haemophilus influenza (especially if not vaccinated)
2. Neisseria meningitis
3. Streptococcal pneumonia

Immunosuppressed patients:
1. Escherichia Coli (Enterics Gram negatives)
2. Listeria Monocytogenes
3. Cryptococcal in Aids patients

Neonate meningitis:
1. Group B Streptococcus
2. Escherichia Coli.

3. Listeria monocytogenes

Neutropenic patients:
1. Pseudomonas Aeruginosa
2. Enterobacteriaceae.

Cryptococcal: Most common fungal meningitis, increased risk factors include exposure to pigeon excrement, & immunosupressed patients. Latex agglutination for cryptococcal antigen is most sensitive marker; India ink stain has high rate of false negatives.
Rx:
1. **Amphotericin B** SE: nephrotoxicity, hypomagnesia, hypokalemia, RTN (renal tubular necrosis) **Check:** magnesium, & K$^+$.
2. +/- **Flucytosine: Check:** LFT, renal function, CBC. SE: myelosuppression.

Escherichia coli: Gram-negative bacillus, immunocompromised & neonates are at increase risk.
Rx:
1. **Ceftriaxone** SE: pseudomembranous colitis, increase in PT/INR due to vitamin K deficiency.
2. & **Gentamicin** SE: nephrotoxicity, ototoxicity, & vestibular.

Haemophilus Influenza: Gram-negative pleomorphic rods, type B capsule; labs media: heme (X)/ NAD (factor V). Typical cases: otitis media, bronchitis, septicemia, epiglottitis, & meningitis in unvaccinated patients. Complications include hearing loss.
Rx: Cefotaxime; if patient not vaccinated consider steroids.

Herpes Simplex Virus (HSV): CSF findings are lymphocytic predominance, increase protein, + RBC, HSV not cultured from the CSF. Diagnosis by (PCR) for herpes DNA in CSF.

Herpes encephalitis: Cowdry type A inclusion body, olfactory or gustatory hallucinations, anosmia, temporal lobe seizures, personality changes, delirium, aphasia, hemiparesis & "Necrotizing Hemorrhagic Encephalitis." CT less sensitive than MRI: temporal lobe inflammation (early diagnosis). Complications of disease include: neurologic deficits, memory disorder, & seizures.

Rx: IV acyclovir SE: crystalluria. (See medications section)

Listeria Monocytogenes: Gram-negative rod, crosses placenta (especially 3rd trimester) newborns at increase risk. Other patients at risk include elderly, diabetics & transplant patients.

S/s: of newborns can present with acute meningitis (rarely), premature delivery or chorioamnionitis. Other infections include gastroenteritis & granulomatous infantisepticum.

Rx:
1. **Ampicillin** with other antibiotic **SE:** eosinophilia, pseudomembranous colitis.
2. **Gentamicin**.

Neisseria Meningitis: Gram-negative diplococcus, patients at increase risk include military, college students (dorms), & C5-C8 deficiency. Transmission is by air borne droplets.

S/s: meningeal symptoms, fever, chills, rash; if severe, patient may have Waterhouse-Friderichsen syndrome. Labs: CSF: Gram neg diplococci, latex agglutination test. Vaccine: YWCA & W135 antigen; this vaccine is limited since it does not cover for B antigen.

Prophylaxis for close contacts use **Rifampin** SE: (see medication section).

Rx:

1. **Penicillin G** SE: seizures, & renal toxicity.
2. **Cefotaxime** SE: Coombs positive, hemolytic anemia.

Waterhouse-Friderichsen: Shock, DIC, bilateral adrenal insufficiency (hemorrhagic necrosis of adrenal glands), petechia found on the trunk & mucous membranes, hypo/hyperpyrexia.
Rx: Steroids. Reverse isolation (protect them from illnesses that others may be carrying).

Streptococcus Pneumonaie: Gram-positive diplococcus, typical case: after blunt head trauma, leakage of CSF, otitis media, & sinusitis. This is the #1 cause of meningitis in adults & asplenic patients.
Rx: Penicillin G, cefotaxime, if penicillin resistant then Vancomycin & ceftriaxone. Prevention: Pneumococcal vaccine especially for high-risk groups: sickle cell, asplenia, & immunosuppressed.

Streptococcal Agalactiae (B): Neonatal meningitis, ↑ risk if baby is born prior to 37 wks gestation or PROM (premature rupture of membranes).

Tuberculous meningitis: Gradual behavioral changes progressing to headache, vomiting, seizures, cranial nerves abnormalities, tuberculosis in other organ & hydrocephalus. CSF: large increase in protein, decrease glucose levels, increased opening pressure, 0-1000 WBC (PMN early, lymphocytes predominate late), CSF C-reactive protein detection & CSF adenosine deaminase. Acid-fast stains, cultures are often negative.
Rx: RIPE: Rifampin SE: red: tears, urine & sweat secretion. **INH:** SE: hepatitis, neuritis (give B6).
Pyrazinamide SE: Gout, increase uric acid levels.
Ethambutol SE: optic neuritis.

Complications of Bacterial Meningitis: Brain edema, seizures, hearing loss, & cranial neuropathies; rare causes include brain abscess, hydrocephalus, & transverse myelitis.

Brain Abscesses: Anaerobes & aerobes, Gram positive cocci, Gram negative rods; if patient is immunocompromised then consider toxoplasmosis. Blood borne infection can result from cardiac (endocarditis), sinusitis, enteric bacteria, Streptococcal (large percentage) & Staphylococcal. The four classic clinical settings include contiguous infection, blood borne infection from distant focus, trauma (staphylococcal) or cryptogenic.
S/s: fever, headache, focal neurologic deficit (hemiparesis) or no symptoms at all.
Dx: by MRI or CT with contrast "ring enhance lesion". Definitive diagnosis is made by needle aspiration or surgical drainage with cultures.
Rx: surgery

(Z): Cysticercus: Associated with travel to South America, South East Asia, & transmission via ingestion of eggs in foods of the pork tapeworm or water that was fecally contaminated. Disease may cause serious nervous damage, headache, vomiting, seizures, ophthalmic damage & space occupying brain lesion.
Dx: punctate calcifications seen on x-ray & CT scan: fluid filled parenchymal cysts. MRI: Ring enhanced cystic lesions.
Rx:
1. **Praziquantel** SE: headaches.
2. Alternative: **Albendazole** SE: leukopenia, hepatotoxic.
3. Test family members stool for tapeworm.

Fungal meningitis:

Rx: Amphotericin B & **fluconazole** enter the CSF adequately. **Ketoconazole** has poor penetration.

(Z): Squire sign: Alternate contraction and dilation of pupil caused by basilar meningitis.

Noninfectious (medications) causes of meningitis:
1. Immunomodulator (IVIG, OKT3 & Cytarabine).
2. NSAIDS
3. Acyclovir & valacyclovir.
4. Antibiotics: gentamicin, amoxicillin & sulfa drugs.

(Z): Vogt-Koyanagi-Harada: Aseptic meningitis, uveitis (small sluggish eye with circumlimbal flush), CN VII damage, alopecia & poliosis. Seen more commonly in Asia compared to US.

Encephalitis: Infection of the parenchyma, meningitis

S/s: disoriented confused, lethargic with difficulty thinking & personality changes.

(Z): Acanthamoeba: Enters via cribriform plate at CN I.

(Z): Naegleria: Lethal meningoencephalitis.

Arthropod-borne Virus: Eastern Equine Encephalitis, St Louis Encephalitis & Western Equine Encephalitis (arbovirus) transmitted by arthropod vectors, mosquitoes, and ticks.
S/s: typically nonspecific with fever, & headache.
Check: CSF: normal glucose, elevated protein. EEG abnormal & serologic testing.
Rx: no specific therapies for arbovirus infections.

BRAIN: FUNCTION & LESIONS

Amygdala: Regulates endocrine activity, sexual behavior, food, H_2O intake. If bilateral damage: **Klüver-Bucy** syndrome: hyperreactivity to visual stimuli, increased oral sexual activity, & disinhibited behavior.

Cerebellar: Check: Dysdiadochokinesia (rapid alternating repetitive motions), past pointing.

Signs of cerebellar lesions: Ataxia, dysarthria, nystagmus, intention, & scanning speech. (Dento-Thalamic tract).

Frontal lobe: Voluntary eye movement; planning & sequencing movement. Lesion to this area can result in inappropriate behavior, disinhibition, deficit with concentration, perseverations, orientation & judgment.

Parietal lobe: Motor control & visual perception. Lesion to the dominant area can cause:
1. Contralateral homonymous hemianopia.
2. Receptive dysphagia
3. Apraxia
4. Gerstmann Syndrome.
5. Spacial neglect syndrome (agnosia of contralateral side from non-dominant side lesion); if dominant hemisphere is affected then alexia, astereognosis & acalculia.

Gerstmann syndrome: Agraphia, acalculia, finger agnosia, right-left disorientation, dyslexia, contralateral: hemianopia (**inferior parietal lesion of dominant lobe).**

Medulla: CN 8-12, audition, cough, vomit, salivation, tongue, respiration & circulation.

Midbrain: CN 3, 4, cerebral aqueduct, loss of upper gaze: pineal area. Ataxia & unstable gait are indicative of posterior fossa involvement.

Occipital: Visual perception, perception of color, movement of objects. Lesions: if unilateral lesion to visual cortex, then "contralateral homonymous hemianopsia" if lesion to visual area with temporal lobe results in the inability to recognize objects & their colors. Other symptoms include hallucinations, visual illusions, & inability to recognize words.

Pons: CN 5-8, Mastication, eye, facial expression, salivation, equilibrium, & audition.

Locked In Syndrome: Ischemic/hemorrhage to Pons, basilar artery occlusion. Paralysis of all cranial nerves is seen except for vertical eye movement. Patient will be able to receive and understand sensory stimuli. Patient will have normal EEG.

Temporal lobe: Auditory & visual perception, learning, emotions. Lesion to this area results in memory & emotion disturbances, Wernicke aphasia, & psychomotor convulsions. Consider (HSV) Herpes simplex virus.

STROKES

Stroke: Signs & symptoms are specific to area of brain that was damaged, persisting for > 5 days & irreversible.
Important to note: the brain is not able to fully autoregulate its blood pressure (BP), especially during the first 10 days following

the stroke. Therefore, discontinue or decrease BP medications gradually; allow BP to be on the high range. Only correct if the diastolic pressure is over 130 mm Hg. Important to fluid restrict.

CT without contrast, rule out hemorrhagic vs. ischemic stroke,70% of strokes (thrombotic 40%, embolic 30%), lacunar 20%, hemorrhagic (10 %). Hemmorrhagic strokes: due to chronic hypertension, patients complain of occipital headaches. If CT is normal & a high index of suspicion, then it is important to order an MRI. **Important to remember** that in the first 12 hrs 50% of CT scans can be normal, this is why strokes are not ruled out in the first 12 hours of a stroke.

Work up of stroke includes chest x-ray, ECG, carotid duplex or transesophageal echocardiography (TEE), Fasting lipid profile, +/-coagulation studies, & MRI (if pathology in the posterior fossa), MRA. If patient is young, evaluate for cocaine use; factor V Leiden, antithrombin III, protein C & S deficiency, homocysteine, lupus panel, ANA & anticardiolipin antibodies. It is important to also consider Moyamoya and Fibromuscular dysplasia. Other tests: CBC, chemistry profile, ESR,

Risk factors for stroke: age, HTN, atherosclerosis, smoking, hyperlipidemia, diabetes, & males.

Amaurosis Fugax: Typical patient will be 50+ year old with transient blindness resulting from a transient ischemia due to ipsilateral carotid artery insufficiency secondary to atheroma, retinal artery embolus, or vessel occluson & pathology.

Medications:

- **Heparin:** IV, SC, rapid onset, mechanism: potentiates

inhibitory action of antithrombin III.

Check PTT. **I**ntrinsic pathway - think of "PITT". Remember that heparin can induce thrombocytopenia. To correct in overdose of heparin, use **Protamine sulfate.**

- **Warfarin**: Oral, K dependent 2, 7,9,10, Protein C & S
  Check: INR, **PT E**xtrinsic PET. Side effects of drug: hemorrhagic complications (purple toes, tissue necrosis especially with hereditary or deficiency of protein C & S. Reversal of warfarin with Vitamin K or rapid reversal with fresh frozen plasma IV.

t-PA: Use within 3hrs of stroke that has a measurable neurologic deficit.
Check CT: Rule out hemorrhage, tumor or mass effect before using tPA. Follow latest hospital guidelines before giving medication.

Exclusion criteria: Recent surgery within the last 14 days, head trauma or stroke with in the last 3 months, seizures at onset of stroke, possible SAH (subarachnoid hemorrhage), persistent systolic BP > 185, or diastolic BP > 110 mm Hg, hypercoagulable state, or heparin, elevated PTT, Glucose <50, or >400.

RIND: **R**eversible **I**schemic **N**eurologic **D**eficit: an ischemic event (i.e. neurological deficit of at least 1 day to 3 days in duration with full recovery); this is an old term, not used.

TIA: Neurological signs & symptoms of vascular nature have sudden onset & last < 24hrs; without headache therefore indicative of an occlusive origin. If severe headache, suspect a hemorrhagic stroke. Remember if 70-99% stenosis of or ulcerated plaques at the carotid bifurcation are found causing occlusion, then surgery is indicated. Patients are at increase risk of having a stroke.

Rx:

1. Antiplatelet: **Aspirin 325 mg**: Important to start within 24 hours of the event in order to prevent second stroke. **Do not use in a hemorrhagic stroke.** Caution with asthmatics. SE: renal, tinnitus, dizziness. If allergic to aspirin, then use other platelet inhibitor.
2. **Ticlopidine**: SE: black box warning, neutropenia, agranulocytosis, TTP, aplastic anemia.
3. **Dipyridamole** SE: dizziness, abdominal discomfort. Consider lipid-lowering drugs;
4. consult physical therapy & occupational therapy.

CIRCLE OF WILLIS SYMPTOMS

Anterior cerebral artery: Contralateral hemiplegia of leg> arm, or behavior changes. If bilateral, then bowel, bladder incontinence; frontal release signs (grasp, suck reflex). This area supplies corpus callosum, basal ganglion, & internal capsule.

Middle cerebral artery: Most commonly involved artery in strokes; symptoms include contra hemiparesis (arm, face > legs), contralateral homonymous hemianopsia, numbness; if on the dominant side: global aphasia (impaired ability to speak, write, & sign); apraxia (impairment of purposeful movement). Anosognosia (neglect - if nondominant is affected). This artery supplies temporal, anterolateral frontal & parietal lobe.

Posterior cerebral Artery: Contralateral hemisensory loss, homonymous hemianopsia, cortical blindness, paralysis of CN 3, memory defects, spontaneous thalamic pain, sudden hemi-ballistic movement. Other symptoms include visual agnosia, alexia & changes in mental status.

Anterior communication Artery: Most common aneurysm; visual defects.

Posterior communication Artery: CN III palsy

Vertebrobasilar artery: Infarction of medulla or pons. Ipsilateral to lesion: CN abnormal; contralateral: weakness & sensory deficits. Complete: Ophthalmoplegia, pupillary constriction, bilateral weakness/or paralysis, dysphagia & dysarthria. Other symptoms include syncope & coma.

Posterior Inferior Cerebellar Artery PICA: Vertigo, nausea, vomiting, nystagmus, tinnitus, & sometimes unilateral deafness; facial weakness & ipsilateral cerebellar ataxia.

(Z): Wallenberg's Syndrome: (lateral medullary syndrome)**:** Thrombosis: dysarthria, dysphagia, staggering gait vestibular nuclei, & vertigo, hypotonia; Horner syndrome on the ipsilateral side, & loss of pain & temperature senses on the opposite side of the body (Spinothalamic).

Lacunar stroke: Small infarct (< 1 cm) of deep penetrating arterioles: at internal capsule, pons, thalamus & basal ganglion; African Americans > Hispanics are at higher risk
Important note: there is no loss of cognition.

S/s:
1. Pure motor hemiplegia (Posterior internal capsule, corona radiate)

2. Pure sensory (thalamus).
3. Ataxic hemiparesis (Pons, Posterior internal capsule or corona radiata)
4. "Dysarthria-clumsy hand" (Pontine) CT can be negative and generally prognosis is good.

Basal Ganglion: Contralateral hemiparesis due to compression of the internal capsule.

Thalamus stroke: Contralateral hemiparesis to stroke: pure hemisensory loss.

Pons: Brain stem dysfunction, "pin point pupils" ophthalmoplegia.

CEREBRAL HEMORRHAGES

Epidural hemorrhage: Mental changes: minutes to hours; occurs between skull & dura; middle meningeal artery damages causes loss of conscious alternating with lucid interval.
S/s: ipsa-lateral dilated pupil (sign of cerebral herniation), hemiparesis contralateral side. Usually patients have temporoparietal fracture.
Test: CT scan of head: deviation of midline structures away from lesion, biconcave (lenticular) shape -extra axial collection of blood.
Rx: emergency surgery: craniotomy & decompression. (For prevention of herniation).

Subarachnoid hemorrhage: Below arachnoid membrane
S/s: sudden headaches, photophobia slow progression, "worst headache of life." projectile vomiting, focal neurologic deficits (VI, hemineglect, memory loss) or coma, increase intracranial pressure; saccular (berry) aneurysms are common cause of bleed. Other

causes include AV malformations.

Test: CT: blood in cisterns, sylvian fissure, ventricles & sulci. LP: bloody (Xanthochromia) tubes 1-4 will all have increase RBC, protein up to 2,000 mg/dL; glucose normal; arteriogram (gold standard) identifies location of lesion.

Rx: raise head of bed; neurosurgery (decompression or clipping the aneurysms); IV mannitol & hyperventilation. Nimodipine: decreases probability of stroke status post subarachnoid hemorrhage by reducing vasospasm. Vasospasms occur in patients with aneurysmal SAH; vasospasms begin 3-5 days post subarachnoid hemorrhage. Give anti seizure medication.

Complications: obstructive hydrocephalus, re-bleed & SIADH.

Subdural: Mental changes in days to weeks; below dura; laceration of bridging veins due to sudden velocity changes causing rapid deterioration. Patients tend to appear sicker & have a higher mortality rate.

Test: LP: xanthochromia; CT: crescent shaped axial collection of blood, usually found contra-coup to the area of injury. Never crosses midline or dural attachments, but will cross suture lines. This condition is also seen in repetitive trauma (boxing & shaken baby syndrome).

PEDIATRICS HEMORRHAGES:

Caput Succedaneum: Edema/blood between skull & scalp extends across suture line. The condition is benign and often self-limiting.

Cephalhematoma: Hemorrhage stops at suture line.

(Z): Subgaleal hematoma: Blood beneath the galea aponeurotica, crosses calvarial sutures. Risk factors include repeated use of vacuum extractor during delivery.

S/s: include periorbital or auricular ecchymosis.

Rx: close observation, scalp pressure dressing, +/- phototherapy.

HERNIATIONS

(Z): Cushing effect: (Cushing triad) Increase in systemic blood pressure, bradycardia, and irregular breathing (hyperventilation) when the intracranial pressure acutely increases second to hemorrhage or mass effect especially in the posterior fossa.

(Z): Central herniation: Decreased mental status; pupillary activity preserved until later in disorder; Cheyne-Stokes respiration (cerebral lesion), followed by decorticate position then a decerebrate posture.

(Z): Tonsillar herniation: Herniation of the cerebellar tonsils through the foramen magnum, causing compression of the medulla that then causes respiratory arrest.

(Z): Uncal herniation: Fixed, dilated pupils due to CN III entrapment, decrease consciousness, & with hemiparesis.

Spinal cord injury protocol: Methylprednisolone 30 mg/kg bolus/1st 30 minutes IV, then 5.4mg/kg/hr next 23hrs.

Severe Head injury: Rx: Hypothermia decreases O_2 demand.

HYDROCEPHALUS

ddx: CMV & Toxoplasmosis, Arnold Chiari malformation & aqueductal stenosis.

Arnold Chiari Malformation:

I: Herniation of the cerebellar tonsils through the foramen magnum, associated with lower CN signs & symptoms: cough, headache. myelomeningocele, syringomyelia.

II: herniation of medulla, tonsil & vermis; associated with spinal/cranial dysraphias. Arnold Chiari is associated with noncommunicating hydrocephalus.

III rare: entire cerebellum with cervico-occipital encephalocele or myelomeningocele.

(Z): Dandy-Walker: Cerebellar vermis is deficient, 4th ventricle enlargement, associated with hydrocephalus.

CSF circulation: Lateral ventricle to interventricular foramento 3rd ventricle to thru cerebral aqueduct of Sylvius 4th ventricle to foramen of Luschka + Magendie to subarachnoid space to arachnoids villi to dural sinus to venous system.

Communicating: Results from inadequate or decrease reabsorption of CSF.

Noncommunicating: Results from obstruction of CSF.

Pediatrics: Check head circumference; ultrasound can be performed if anterior fontanel is patent.

SPEECH

Aphasia: Absence or impairment of ability to communicate through speech, writing, or sign language because of dysfunction of dominant brain hemisphere implying a cortical lesion.

The two most tested are Brocas & Wenicke:

- **Broca's (Motor):** Nonfluent aphasia, decreased rate, decreased phrase length, but good comprehension, no repetition; the lesion is in the dominant frontal lobe. Also known as **Expressive type:** patient cannot express emotion. Patient is aware of deficit.

- **Wernicke: (Sensory)** also known as **Receptive type:** patient cannot understand emotion. Fluent aphasia, with empty content impairment in the comprehension, no repetition, cannot follow instructions. The lesion is in the dominant temporal lobe originating in the left inferior portion of the middle cerebral artery. Patient is not aware of deficit.

OTHER DEFINITIONS & SPEECH PATHOLOGY:

Aphonia: loss of the voice due to disease or injury to the larynx

(Z): Bulbar dysfunction: muscle innervated by the cranial nerves whose nuclei are in the medulla.

Conduction aphasia: poor repetition with good speech & comprehension. Arcuate Fasciculus connects Broca's & Wernicke.

Dysarthria: difficult & defective speech due to impairment of the tongue. Inability to speak even though no defect in ability to understand; defect is in brain stem or cerebellar.

Dysphonia: altered voice production.

Dysphagia: inability to swallow.

Dysprosody: non-dominant hemisphere: language deficient.

(Z): Global aphasia: dominant hemisphere: neither speaks, comprehends, nor repeats words.

(Z): Transcortical sensory aphasia: like Wernicke's but with preserved repetition. The lesion is in the posterior parieto-occipital area.

(Z): Transcortical motor aphasia: Broca's but with preserved repetition (Incomplete Broca's).

DEMYELINATION DISEASE

Central Pontine myelinolysis: Rapid correction of hyponatremia causes demyelination. It is important to correct hyponatremia at a rate of < 0 .5 mEq/L/hr in order to avoid this condition.

ddx: Locked In Syndrome, multiple sclerosis, subarachnoid or cerebellar hemorrhage.

Guillain-Barré Syndrome (GBS): is an example of an **A**cute **I**nflammatory **D**emyelinating **P**olyradiculoneuropathy (AIDP) involving motor function; patient will have ascending weakness, respiratory paralysis, autonomic dysfunction, +/- sensory involvement, decreased /Absent DTR & CN: 6 & 7. *Campylobacter Jejuni* is most commonly identified precipitant of GBS.
Other causes include viral illness, (Cytomegalovirus 2nd most common cause, Epstein-Barr Virus), & history of recent vaccinations.
Test: CSF: albumin-cytologic dissociation; increase protein (>50), normal cell count, & glucose.
Check: EMG, & nerve conduction study (will have slow nerve

conduction late in disease process) & prolonged F-wave latencies (early in disease).

Rx: supportive, plasmapheresis, & IVIG.

Miller Fisher variant of GBS: ataxia, areflexia, ophthalmoplegia, & polyneuropathy. IgG anti-GQ$_{1b}$ antibodies.

ddx: Chronic inflammatory demyelination, HIV, diphtheria, & acute intermittent porphyria.

Chronic Inflammatory Demyelinating Polyradiculoneuropathy (CIDP): Peak incidence is 40-60 years of age. The demyelinating disorder of peripheral nerves can be symmetric sensorimotor disorder. First affecting distal limbs and less often CN, if any usually CN 6 & 7; decrease /absent DTR. Classically, it is chronically progressive or relapsing stepwise progressive with symptoms usually lasting 12 weeks to a year. This can be considered the chronic equivalent of Guillain-Barré Syndrome.

Labs: CSF: cytoalbuminologic dissociation; elevated protein 50-200 mg/dL, mild lymphocytic pleocytosis & gamma globunin levels elevated (associated with HIV). CBC, sedimentation rate, ANA, immunoelectrophoresis serum and urine, EMG, Sural nerve biopsy can aid in diagnosising of CIDP.

Rx: plasmapheresis, prednisone, gabapentin for neuropathic pain.

(Z): Marchiafava-Bignami Syndrome: Symmetric demyelination of corpus callosum; & white matter secondary to alcoholism causing dementia & seizures.

Multiple Sclerosis: Female: 20-40, temperate climate, chronic central degeneration; Charcot's triad: nystagmus, tremor, & scanning speech. Patients have ataxia, weakness, fatigue, visual loss, neuritis, & sexual dysfunction. Condition worsens with heat known as

Uhthoff Phenomenon, double vision with lateral gauze (bilateral internuclear ophthalmoplegia).

Test: MRI: multiple diffuse plaques typically found in periventricular white matter, corpus callosum; sagittal images: show "Dawson fingers." Magnetic resonance spectroscopy helps estimate axonal loss. LP: Oligoclonal bands, IgG, increase myelin basic protein.

Rx:

1. **β Interferon 1a** (Avonex) SE: depression, suicidal ideations, hepatotoxicity & leukopenia,

2. **Glatiramer acetate** (Copaxone) SE**:** chest pain, dyspnea, & palpitations.

3. Chronic: **Azathioprine. Check**: CBC + platelets SE: bone marrow suppression, teratogenic, & hepatotoxicity.

4. **Cyclophosphamide** SE: SIADH, bone marrow suppression & hemorrhagic cystitis. **Check:** WBC/Platelets.

5. **Muscle relaxer**: **Baclofen** (Lioresal) SE: hypotension, sedation, weakness & urinary frequency. If abruptly withdrawn then may have seizures & hallucinations.

6. **Urinary problems**: **Oxybutynin** (Ditropan).

7. **Mitoxantrone** (Novantrone): used for progressively relapsing or worsening of multiple sclerosis. SE: **black box warning** severe local tissue extravasation, abnormal ECG, cardiotoxicity, & bone marrow suppression.

8. **β interferon-1b** (Betaseron) SE: flu like symptoms, hepatotoxicity & leucopenia.

9. **Natalizumab monoclonal antibody** SE: infections, depression joint pain.

NEUROMUSCULAR JUNCTIONS DISEASES & TOXINS

Fatigue, weakness, normal/ decrease DTR.

(Z): α-Bungarotoxins: Blocks acetylcholine receptor (IRR) to nicotinic receptors.

Black Widow: ↑ release of acetylcholine.
 S/s: chest pain, dyspnea, headaches, paresthesia, seizures.
 Rx: cold compresses, steroids, if critical then use Antivenom.
 Check: skin test before dosing Antivenom.

Botulism: The toxin (A > E > B in order of from highest to lowest mortality rate); irreversible; inhibits acetylcholine release from the presynaptic terminals.
 S/s: sudden onset, 12-36hrs, CN palsies (extra ocular movements), **D**ry mouth & eyes, **D**ilated pupils, **D**iplopia, **D**escending paralysis of caudal cranial nerves that cause **D**ysarthria & **D**ysphagia.

The typical case is of an infant ingesting honey, followed by constipation, flaccid paralysis, and weak cry. Disease may progress to respiratory depression. Other risk factors include home canned food.

Check: EMG, cultures & skin test for allergies to horse serum sensitivity prior to administration of antitoxin.
 Rx: antitoxin +/- intubation, antibiotics contraindicated because of the lysis of the organism causes an increase in toxins.
 Prophylaxis: Pentavalent toxoid vaccine (types A, B, C, D, and E) is available as an IND product for those at high risk of exposure.

Myasthenia Gravis: Female>male, mechanism: antibody against postsynaptic acetylcholine receptors

S/s: ptosis & diplopia in 50% patients, fatigue, & limb weakness. Symptoms increase as day progresses. No pupil involvement; patients are at increase risk of thymoma. Aminoglycosides may exacerbate myasthenia gravis. (Note: if diplopia, ptosis, 3rd CN palsy with papillary sparing is suggestive of diabetic cranial mononeuropathy.

Tensilon test: Edrophonium Chloride SE: cholinergic crisis: bradycardia, laryngospasm. The test will cause a rapid reversal of signs & symptoms of myasthenia gravis. If cholinergic crisis occurs, have **atropine** readily available.

Check: Repetitive nerve stimulation test by EMG will show a decrease response. Check for antibody to acetylcholine receptors. In general, physicians should have higher suspicion for other autoimmune disease (Systemic Lupus Erythematosus & Rheumatoid Arthritis).

Pregnancy: Antibody may cross placenta causing the baby to have a transient myasthenia.

Transient Myasthenia Gravis in the neonate: Infants present with generalized hypotonia, respiratory difficulty.

Rx: Pyridostigmine (Mestinon) SE: cholinergic toxicity, bronchospasm, hypersalivation & miosis. Other therapy includes Thymectomy.

Long term Rx: Azathioprine (Imuran) SE: bone marrow suppression, hepatotoxicity, & steatorrhea. Other therapies include (corticosteroids) **Prednisone** SE: psychosis, osteoporosis & hyperglycemia.

Acute Rx: Plasmapheresis + IVIG. Thymectomy may help.

(Z): Ocular myasthenia: Diplopia & ptosis.

(Z): Bilateral Ptosis: Should suspect a midbrain lesion.

(Z): Diabetic mononeuropathy: can affect the cranial nerves of the eyes.

Lambert-Eaton: Muscle weaknesses improve with exercise, decrease/absent DTR and has no eye involvement. EMG improves with increased response. Also, suspect small cell carcinoma (Oat cell); affects the release of acetylcholine via antibody against presynaptic calcium channels in axial muscles. Disease associated with the elderly & long history of smoking.
Rx: treat underling cause, steroids & plasmapheresis.

Tetanus toxin: *Clostridium Tetani*, Gram-negative Rod, spore forming anaerobic producing a neurotoxin that inhibits Renshaw cell release. Symptoms include painful muscular contractions of jaw & neck
Rx: clean wound, & debride, Tetanus vaccine +/- immunoglobulins.

SEIZURES

Make sure to ask patients of events prior, during, status post seizure from patient & observers. Rule out other causes and obtain a CBC, electrolyte, Ca++, Mg++, NH_4, glucose, arterial blood gas, liver function tests, renal tests, TSH, RPR, drug toxicity screen, seizure medication levels, ETOH,(video) EEG, & MRI. Seizures can commonly cause posterior shoulder dislocation.

Seizures: Attacks are of sudden onset.

Epilepsy: Chronic disorder, paroxysmal brain dysfunction secondary to increased neuronal discharge usually associated with some alteration of consciousness.

Driver's license taken away until patient is disease free for months to years depending on which state (Texas: 6 months).

ddx for seizure: Hypoglycemia, migraine, paroxysmal vertigo, vasovagal syncope, TIA, breath holding spells, pseudoseizures & narcolepsy.

Pseudoseizure:

Check: psychiatric history and EEG (normal); can often be seen with patients that truly have seizures (patient malingering).

Partial: one area of brain.

Rx: phenytoin, carbamazepine.

Simple Partial (focal): only one part of the hemisphere (cerebral cortex) is affected, so no loss of conscious (LOC).

Motor jerking body part (Jacksonian March), **sensory** (tingling of body part), autonomic (abd/epigastric sensation), psychologic, memory & emotional disturbances (lasts seconds). During the postictal phase, patient can have Todd's paralysis.

EEG: spikes & sharp waves.

Todd's paralysis: Transient postictal hemiparesis status post focal seizures lasting up to 24 hrs.

Complex Partial: (psychomotor):Most common seizure, Male in 1st & 6th decade of life.

S/s: altered taste, smell, auditory, visual hallucinations, déjà vu or jamais vu, altered consciousness (awake but not aware of surroundin*g)* & **amnesia**. Other symptoms include **A**utomatisms, chewing, & lip smacking; symptoms can last from 30 seconds to several minutes.

Check: EEG (interictal spikes), MRI (temporal lobe) & no loss of conscious.

Rx: Phenytoin/Tegretol.

Generalized: Entire area of brain is affected at once causing tonic-clonic seizures with loss of conscious.

Grand Mal: Generalized Tonic Clonic (GTC): (↑ serum prolactin), unconsciousness, convulsions, muscle rigidity, complex generalized tonic-clonic seizures. Incontinence, tongue lacerations & postictal state (confused & headache). Usually lasts 1-3 minutes. **Tonic:** Muscle stiffness, rigidity.

Rx: Valproic acid .

Clonic: Repetitive, rhythmic jerking movements.

Myoclonic: Sporadic, sudden isolated jerking movements.

Atonic: Loss of muscle tone, leads to falls ("drop attack"), typically seen in infant/kids that causes injury.

Status Epilepticus: Seizures for 30 minutes or greater or recurrent seizures without recovery of consciousness in between. True emergency, morbidity, and mortality correlate with the time in status epilepticus with permanent neuronal injury ocurring after 1 hour of continous seizure.

Check: electrolytes, glucose, medications levels & obtain history of compliance with medications. Other common causes include alcohol withdrawal, metabolic abnormality, brain tumor &

cerebral infarction.

Rx:

1. ABC, check glucose, electrolytes, anticonvulsant levels, drug screen toxicity, EEG, & EKG.

2. IV **Lorazepam**: SE: cardiovascular collapse, respiratory depression, paradoxical CNS stimulation. or **Diazepam**: SE: respiratory depression, tinnitus, blurred vision. (Consider vitamin B1 & dextrose).
   If refractory: +/- **Phenytoin** (fosphenytoin).
   If still refractory, give **Phenobarbital** SE: sedative, blood dyscrasias, angioedema, and paradoxical CNS stimulation.

INFANTS/CHILDREN/OBSTETRICS

Absence (petit mal): EEG: 3-3.5 HZ spike & slow waves. Before age 10 years of age, symptoms include staring, distracted, loss of posture, chewing, usually last >15 seconds.
Important to note that there is no post ictal phase. Seizures can be elicited by hyperventilating the patient for 3 minutes.
Rx: (without tonic clonic): **Ethosuximide** SE: Steven Johnson syndrome, blood dyscrasias. (With tonic clonic): **Valproate**. Brief LOC. Diet: medium chain triglyceride diet.

Breath holding spells: Ages 18 months to 3 years, typically provoked by an event that makes the child upset.
Two types: cyanotic & pallid spells.
Blue spells, cyanotic spells precipitated by upsetting situation. The child screams loudly then becomes noiseless as child holds breath for 20-30 seconds. The entire episode usually lasts less than one minute. Pale spells follow a fearful or painful experience. Begin to suspect seizures if patient does not have a precipitating event, no history of crying or holding breath, episode last > 1 minute, the

age is not typical of breath holding spells.

Rx: parental support and reassurance, usually resolves by the time the child is 4-5 years old.

(Z): Benign Rolandic brief epilepsy: Infrequent, brief facial; most twitches occurring at the transitions between wakefulness & sleep, usually affects previously healthy children ages 5-12 years old. EEG: Rolandic area spikes, centrotemporal spikes.

Rx: Carbamazepine. Most seizures abate after puberty.

Eclampsia: Seizure or coma unrelated to other cerebral conditions often occurs in the third trimester of pregnancy or within the first 48 hours status post delivery. If patient has eclampsia prior to 20 weeks, suspect molar pregnancy or antiphospholipid syndrome. This condition can occur upto 3 weeks after delivery.

Rx: delivery of the fetus and placenta is the only curative treatment.

Febrile Seizures: are due to the rapid rise in temperature. Simple seizures (<15mins) or 1x seizure/24hrs; complex >15 minutes or >1 seizures/24hrs. Disease is seen ages 5 months to 5 years peaks during 14-18 months. Rapid rise of temperature > 102 F, generalized tonic-clonic in simple seizures and focal seizures in complex. Normal EEG & negative family history of seizures; the recurrent rates are 50% in 6 months, 75% in 1 year and 90% will recur in 2 years. This condition can be seen with Roseola infantum. If child under 18 months of age or cannot find source of fever, consider Lumbar puncture.

Rx: treat underlying cause of fever (URI, acute otitis media, etc) & use age appropriate antipyretics. **Phenobarbital, phenytoin, & carbamazepine** have not been shown to reduce reoccurrence. Diazepam can help if given immediately at the onset of fever.

(Z): Infantile spasms: Generalized seizures involving flexor spasms of the extremities & trunk, hypsarrhythmia (EEG), developmental regression or delay (mental retardation) are consistent with **West Syndrome**; underlying brain disease originating from pre (peri) post natal causes (Tuberous sclerosis, PKU) which affects ages 4 months to 8 months. These children at increase risk for developing **Lennox-Gastaut syndrome** (child onset epilepsy, often seen in patients with mental retardation and behavior problems) more information below.

Check: EEG, MRI & CT.

Rx: ACTH SE: hypertension, glucose intolerance, cardiac failure & gastric hemorrhage. Other treatments: **clonazepam**, **valproic acid** (helps myoclonus), **ketogenic diet** or **prednisone** depending on cause of infantile spasms.

(Z): Juvenile Myoclonic epilepsy: Adolescence female with normal intelligence, early morning myoclonic seizures arms > legs which can be precipitated by lack of sleep; lesions can be found on chromosome 6, autosomal dominant. EEG: 4-6 Hz polyspike & wave

Rx:
1. **Valproic acid SE: Weight gain, check liver function.**
2. **Primidone SE:** vertigo & coordination problems.
3. **Lamotrigine SE:** headaches.

(Z): Lennox-Gastaut Syndrome: Myoclonic astatic epilepsy in children with mental retardation, multiple seizure types (generalized tonic, atonic, myoclonic, tonic-clonic, & atypical absence seizures); poor prognosis. EEG: slow 1-2 Hz spike & wave.

Rx: **1. Valproic acid 2. Felbatol** SE: aplastic anemia & fatal hepatic failure.

Neonate seizures: Symptoms include repetitive eye blinking, tonic or clonic movement of single extremity & apnea.
Check: Glucose & calcium can be low in gestational diabetes & inpreterm infants; obtain magnesium levels should be evaluated; obtain a more detailed history (mother drug dependent). Other etiologies include hypoxic ischemic encephalopathy, intracranial hemorrhage, CNS infection, & pyridoxine deficiency.
Rx: treat underlying cause, **phenobarbital** SE: hypotension, & respiratory failure.

Shigellosis: Gram-negative bacilli; neurologic signs & symptoms include seizures, altered mental status, especially in children.
Rx: **Bactrim**. If patient is allergic then use **Azithromycin**.

OTHER CAUSES:

Hyperthyroidism: Fingers spread apart, arms extended, flexion & extension in a static kinetic tremor.

Medications Associated with Seizures: Carbonmonoxide, Bupropion, Cefepime, Ganciclovir, Levaquin, tetracycline, cyclosporin & anesthetics.

OD: INH, Salicylate, Theophylline, Lithium & Cocaine.

Thallium poisoning: seizure, GI s/s, headache & primarily sensory involvement.

MEDICATIONS OF ANTIEPILEPTIC/SIDE EFFECT

NOTE: Treatment should not begin until patient has had 2nd seizures or more. In females, check β-HCG before giving antiepileptic medications.

Carbamazepine (Tegretol): therapeutic range: 4-12 mcg/ml
SE: aplastic anemia, SIADH, Steven Johnson's syndrome, hyponatremia, pancytopenia, anticholinergic effects; may interfere with oral contraceptive, hepatotoxicity.
Check: CBC q wk for 2 months then q3 weeks, liver function test Q3 month; serum therapeutic levels are 4-10 μg/mL.

Ethosuximide (Zarontin) SE: Ataxia, Vascular +/- drug induced lupus, pancytopenia, abnormal liver function test, serum therapeutic levels 40-100 μg/ml.
Check: CBC & liver functions q6 months.

Fe*lb*amate: SE: *Liver + Bone Marrow toxicity.*

Fosphenytoin SE: Perineal itching, serum: 5-20 μg/ml

Gabapentin (Neurontin) SE: Behavior changes, dizziness, nystagmus, amnesia, tremor, leucopenia, & weight gain.

Lamotrigine (Lamictal) SE: Steven-Johnson syndrome, Toxic Epidermal Necrolysis, aplastic anemia, diplopia, & ataxia.

Phenytoin (Dilantin) Do not use in 2nd or 3rd degree heart block, SE: Gingival hyperplasia, hirsutism, lupus-like, agranulocytosis, megaloblastic anemia, osteomalacia, arrhythmia, osteoporosis, cerebellar ataxia, pleural effusions, interferes with OCP. Serum levels should be between 5-20 µg/ml

Check: Ca^{2+}, ataxia & nystagmus (gazed evoked).

Topiramate (Topamax) SE: renal stones, memory difficulty, angle closure glaucoma, aphasia hyperchloremic, non-anion gap metabolic acidosis, & ataxia.

Valproic acid (Depakene) SE: Hepatotoxicity, bleeding tendency, thinning hair, tremor, weight gain, ankle edema, pancreatitis, neutropenia, neural tube defects. Serum 50-150 µg/ml.

Check: liver function tests q 6mo, CBC, platelet count q 3mo. Serum amylase q3 months.

Other antiseizure medications:

Clonazepam (Klonopin) SE: respiratory depression, memory impairment, depression, & dry mouth.

Levetiracetam SE: leukopenia, asthenia & ataxia.

Tiagabine SE: Steven Johnson's syndrome, confusion.

Zonisamide (Zonegran) {sulfonamide} SE: Steven Johnson's Syndrome, agranulocytosis, & aplastic anemia.

Treatment for intractable seizures:
1. Surgery: temporal lobectomy
2. Vagus nerve stimulator.

Pregnancy & Seizure patients: Continue seizure medications, + or − decreasing the dose.

Check: medication levels especially in 3rd trimester; check for neural tube defects, increase folic acid vitamins (4 mg/day) 3 months prior to pregnancy. Breast-feeding is permitted.

Anti-epileptic drugs & potential fetal/neonatal effects:
1. **Carbamazepine**: spina bifida.
2. **Phenobarbital**: orofacial clefts, cardiac malformations & impaired cognitive performance.
3. **Phenytoin**: orofacial clefts, cardiac & urogenital malformations.
4. **Valproate:** Neurotubal defects(meningomyelocele), cardiovascular & urogenital malformations.

Neural Tube Defects:
1. **Spinal bifida occulta**: midline defect of vertebral bodies, no protrusion of spinal contents; no external sac.
   Check: for dimpling, lipoma, & hairy patch.
2. **Meningocele**: midline defect of vertebral arches. The spinal cord does not herniate, but the meninges do herniate. Patients are at increase risk of syringomyelia.
3. **Meningomyelocele**: more frequent defect, posterior defect & herniation of meninges and neural tissue. Increase risk of having Chiari malformation, seizures, & neurologic deficit depending on level of malformation.
4. **Rachischisis**: embryologic failure of fusion of vertebral arches & posterior neural tube.

TUMORS

Adults: supratentorial
Kids: infratentorial

Astrocytoma: overall it is the 2ⁿᵈ most common and the most common type of tumor in the posterior fossa of children. Patients complain of morning headache. This type of tumor is a low-grade malignancy with slow growth; May have symptoms of paralyzes of CN 5, 7, 10 unilaterally. Think of it as "**C**ystic Astrocytoma: **C**hildren **C**erebellum".
Rx: surgical excision & radiation.

Glioblastoma multiforme: Most common malignant tumor in adults. It is a Grade 4 Astrocytoma with rapid growth. It can be fatal. In the elderly; tumor crosses midline via the corpus collasum, found in frontal, temporal, & basal ganglion. Pathology: pseudopalisading arrangement of tumor cells.

Meningioma: 2ⁿᵈ most common benign tumor in adults, from dura matter, & arachnoid. Pathology slides "psammoma bodies" located inparasagittal area, falx cerebri, sphenoidal ridge, & olfactory groove; female > male ages 40s & 70s; associated with neurofibromatosis II, not invasive hyperostosis. Tumor can be seen on MRI with contrast or CT scan. This disease has a good prognosis.

Ependymoma: Benign, perivascular pseudorosettes. Often causes a communicating hydrocephalus resulting from the obstruction of the 4th ventricle seen mostly in children.

Medulloblastoma: Is the most common malignant brain tumor of childhood.
S/s: headache, ataxic, projectile vomit & nausea, focal neurologic signs & symptoms such as ataxia. Tumor arises from the floor of 4th ventricle causing blockage of CSF which then increases ICP, hydrocephalus. Most common neoplasm of posterior fossa in

young kids ages 2 to 10 years of age male>female, MRI: midline cerebellar mass. Malignant tumor of cerebellar (pseudorosette) origin that then metastasizes to bone.
Rx: radiosensitive, chemotherapy, & surgery.

Craniopharyngioma: (Rathke pouch tumor). Calcified cystic slow-growing tumor supratentorial is a cause of short stature, delay in puberty, diabetes insipidus
S/s: hypothyroidism, visual changes, hypogonadism, & headaches. Adult male complain of impotence; female complain of amenorrhea. The CT scan with & without contrast demonstrates a (supra) sellar calcified cyst. Plain skull radiographs can also show calcifications & increase Prolactin levels.
Rx: hormone replacement therapy, needle aspiration & surgery.

Neuroblastoma: Anywhere along neural crest cells adrenal medulla, cervical- thoracic sympathetic chain, ↑ vanillylmandelic acid (VMA).
Check: for N-myc oncogene.

Mets to brain: Usually from Lungs> breast>GI to white grey junction. Others from: Lymphoma, melanoma, renal.

DERMATOMES

C4: **above collarbone**
C7: **middle finger**
T4: **Nipple line**
T7: **xiphoid process.**
T10: **umbilicus**
L5: **lateral leg-big toe**

S3: **Anus**

S2-S4: **Lateral foot/saddle area**

C3, C4, C5 keeps the diaphragm alive.

Biceps: C5-C6 (Musculocutaneous).

Brachioradial (supinator): C5-C6 (Radial).

Triceps: C6-C8 (Radial).

Patellar: L2-L4 (Femoral).

Achilles: L5-S2, (Tibial)

Plantar: L4-S2.

Cremaster: L1-L2 (elevates testicles/scrotum).

Bulbocavernosus reflex: S3-S4 (male: squeeze base of penis, observe contraction of anal sphincter. This reflex is absent in sacral cord disease.

Anal reflex: S2-S5.

S2, S3, S4: keeps the feces off the ground.

DEEP TENDON REFLEXES

0 = absent reflex

1+ = trace, hyporeflexic (no joint movement)

2+ = normal

3+ = hyperreflexic (brisk) without clonus

4+ = 1-3 beats of clonus with contralateral reflex,

5+ = strong contraction, sustained clonus, spread contralateral reflex.

Delayed relaxation phase of deep tendon reflexes ddx: hypothyroid, pernicious anemia, diabetes, & Parkinson.

Hyporeflexic: Tabes dorsalis, poliomyelitis, myasthenia gravis, hemorrhage, diabetes mellitus, CNS depressing & medications.

Hyperreflexic: Corticospinal lesion, UMN, pyramidal lesion, & thyrotoxicosis.

(Z): Pendular reflex: knee jerk continues to swing due to cerebellar lesion.

HANDS & ARMS:

- **Radial**: C5-8: **Check** extend thumb. Typical cases: fracture of spiral groove of humerus, Saturday night palsy, lead poisoning: painless neuropathy: wrist drop. Other nerve specific symptoms include sensory loss on dorsal aspect of hand.

- **Ulnar**: C8-T1: **Check** adduction of thumb, Trauma to ulnar grove at elbow can present with numbness of 5th digit and medial 4th digit, clawhand and atrophy or weakness of thumb adductor, & interossi.

- **Median**: C5-T1 **Check** opposition of thumb

- **Musculocutaneus**: C5, 6 Fracture of humerus: can damage the biceps & coracobrachialis.

- **Axillary Nerve:** Anterior Glenohumeral dislocation.

LEGS:

- **Femoral (L2-L4)** loss of knee jerk.

- **Obturator (L2-L4)**: cannot adduct hip.

- **Sciatic nerve:** fracture of acetabulum.

- **Common Peroneal (L2-L4)**: foot drop, absent eversion or dorsiflexion, "toes drag when walking," "slapping" gait.

- **Tibial (L4-S3):** loss of plantar flexion, absent inversion/plantar flexion.

- **Carpal tunnel**: median nerve entrapped. Thenar atrophy,

weak grip, decreases sensation of first 3 ½ lateral digits.
Check: Phalen, Tinel signs, direct (carpel) compression test, electromyography (EMG) & nerve conduction studies this condition worsens with pregnancy due to increase edema.
Rx: NSAIDS, wrist splint & surgical decompression.

Phalen's test: (the exam looks like the patient is handcuffed like a felon)**:** flex wrist; wait 1-minute: causes paresthesia in a median nerve distribution.

Tinel's Sign: Tapping radial side of palmaris longus **T**endon causes **T**ingling indicative of carpal **T**unnel.

Cervical rib (Thoracic Outlet Syndrome): Compression of inferior brachial plexus: commonly C8 & T1 due to rib or neck trauma; symptoms include atrophy of interosseous, thenar, hypothenar muscles. Sensory deficit of forearm, hand usually in ulnar distribution; decrease radial pulse when head is moved to opposite side. Cervical rib (extra rib) arises from C7 vertebra.
Check: cervical x-ray, EMG, color duplex Doppler, CT scan or MRI with angiography.
Rx: underlying cause, physical therapy & surgical.

Erb-Duchenne palsy: Tear at **C5-C6** roots, "waiters tips"

Kl*U*mpke palsy: Lesion to lower trunk of brachial plexus, C8- T1, claw hand, ulnar nerve. Patient may have trouble spreading fingers. Nerve is typically injured during birth due to shoulder dystocia.

Mononeuritis multiplex: Nontraumatic involvement of the peripheral nervous system (roots, nerve trunks),
Check: nerve biopsy, nerve conduction studies: axonal damage.

ddx: often as a result of vasculitides, other causes include DM, trauma, rheumatoid arthritis, sarcoidosis, tumor, HIV, Lyme disease & Leprosy.
Rx: corticosteroids.

Nursemaid elbow: Subluxation of radial head from the annular ligament caused by sudden traction on the hand with the elbow extended and the forearm pronated. Normal x-rays, the diagnosis is by history & physical.
Rx: forceful supinating with forearm extended followed by flexion of the forearm.

(Z): Reflex sympathetic dystrophy: Painful neuropathic signs & symptoms status post trauma or surgery.
Stage I: Acute stage: burning, hyperalgesia, ↑ hair & nail growth.
Stage II: Dystrophic stage: muscle tremors & spasms, ↑ muscle tone/DTR, hair loss, brittle nails, x-ray may show osteoporosis.
Stage III: Atrophy stage: cold, fixed joints, contractures & irreversible tissue damage.

Wing Scapula: Long thoracic nerve damage due to mastectomy.

CLASSIC SIGNS/TESTS

Allen: Occlude both radial/ulnar artery & access for blood flow.

Arcus Senilis: An opaque, grayish ring at the periphery of the cornea, seen in elderly.

Babinski: Dorsiflexion of great toe, fanning of the other toes (lesion in pyramidal tract above L4). Normal response is flexion of all the toes.

Battle: Discoloration in the line of posterior auricular artery ecchymosis of mastoid process indicative of basilar skull fracture.

Café Au Lait Spots: Pigmented cutaneous lesions, ranging from light to dark brown, neurofibromatosis I (von Recklinghausen disease).

Chaddock's Reflex: Stimulate lateral foot, extension of the great toe then corticospinal reflex paths (alt to Babinski).

Chvostek: Facial spasm via tapping CN 7th indicative of hypocalcemia.

Coordination: Finger to nose, heel to shin.

Clonus (UMN): Spasmodic alternation of muscular contractions between antagonistic muscle groups caused by a hyperactive stretch reflex.

Coma: Unconsciousness that is reversible (no response to sound, light or deep pain).
ddx: Alcoholism/**A**bscess, **E**ncephalopathy/**E**pidural hematoma, **I**nsulin decrease/ increase **I**schemic/ **I**nfection/**I**nflammation (vasculitis), **O**piates/hyp**o**xia/hyp**o**natremia, **U**remia/metabolic disorder, trauma, stroke, shock, poisoning, psychiatric disorder (malignant catatonia).
Rx: ABC, dextrose, O2, naloxone, thiamine. Mneumonic (DON'T)

Brain death: Cessation and irreversibility of all brain function, including brain stem.

Brain stem death criteria:

Test:
1. Pupillary response
2. Cornea response
3. Vestibular-ocular reflex
4. Motor response in C.N distributions
5. Gag/tracheal response
6. Respiratory response to hypercapnia (pCO2> 60)
7. No EEG required. No sedatives or hypnotics can be present (absence of endogenous or exogenous toxins). Patient is unresponsive, irreversible lesion or event. It is important to know the nature of coma.

DecorticAte: Extension of leg, flexion of arms, lesion above red nucleus, often diencephalon, thalamic lesion. Decorticate position is a higher mental function than decerebrate.

DEcErEBRatE: (Extensor) posturing: Uninhibited **E**xtension of all **4** **E**xtremities, seen with lesion to midbrain, **B**elow **R**ed nucleus but above vestibular nucleus.

Dolls eye (Oculocephalic reflex) : Dissociation between head & eyes indicative of global diffuse disorder of cerebrum. Do not perform if you suspect cervical injury.

Dysmetria: Inability to control distance, power, & speed. Patients have irregular, jerky movements.

Grasp Reflex: Ask patient to hold finger & let go. If patient does not let go, this is indicative of frontal or encephalopathy lesion.

Glabellar reflex: Percusses glabellar (7th CN) causes constant blinking of eyes caused by UMN lesion or frontal lobe origin.

(Z): Hoffmann's Sign: Support patient's hand & flex the distal phalangeal joint of the middle finger, then quickly release the flexed phalanx & observe for flexion of the terminal phalanx of the thumb. Positive sign may be indicative of (UMN), unilaterally Pyramidal Tract Disease, corticospinal tract, or frontal lobe lesion. This test is equivalent to Babinski sign.

(Z): Lasègue sign: Hip flexed & knee extended, dorsiflexion of the ankle causing pain or muscle spasm in the posterior thigh in affected side probable disk herniation, dorsal column tract lesion, & sciatica).

Lhermitte sign: Sudden electric-like shocks extending down the spine on flexing the head. Non-specific sign seen in multiple sclerosis, tumor, & herniated disc.

Moro reflex: Evoked by loud sound & sudden extension of the neck or limbs; normal response until 4 to 5 months of age.

(Z): Oppenheim reflex: Thumb/index finger down medial tibia causes fanning of the toes; indicates UMN. This is an alternative to the Babinski test.

(Z): Patrick's Test: FABERE (**F**lexion, **A**bduction, **E**xt. **R**otation, & **E**xtension causes pain in patients with hip joint disease or sacroiliitis disease (Ankylosing spondylitis).

Pronator drift: Close eyes; ask patient to put arms out parallel to floor with palms up, observe for pronation. If patient pronates one arm & drifts downward, this is indicative of weakness on one side. If both arms drift down, then suspect bilateral weakness. If arms rise, then suspect cerebellar disease or loss of position (sense especially if patient is searching or having writhing movements). Finally, if one forearm pronates, then suspect contralateral lesion in corticospinal tract.

(Z): Radovici sign: Scratching thenar imminence causes palmomental primitive reflex: ipsilateral contraction of muscle of chin due to corticospinal tract lesion second to increase ICP.

Romberg's Sign: Feet together, patient stands with eyes open & then closed; if closing the eyes causes decrease balance, this is indicative of a loss of proprioceptive (dorsal column function) and midline cerebellar function
ddx: tabes dorsales & labyrinthine disorder).

Setting Sun sign: Downward deviation of eyes, iris "sets" beneath lower eyelid indicative of increase ICP, or irritation of brain stem.

Snout reflex: 7th CN: percussion of the upper lip at midline region of philtrum causes brief puckering of the lips in UMN or frontal lobe lesions. This is considered to be a primitive reflex.

Straight leg raise: Can also illicit (Lasègue sign) by dorsiflexion of the foot when raising leg; the patient supine, pain results from leg being elevated with knee extended; relieved by knee flexion causes sciatic/root nerve irritation L4-S3. Pain in the opposite side known as the crossed leg (opposite leg) response may indicate disk bulge medial to the opposite side root.

(Z): Titubation: Shaking tremor of trunk "head", stagger gait, indicative of cerebellar lesion.

Whipple triad in Insulinoma:

1. Symptoms of hypoglycemia
2. CNS dysfunction that is reversible with administration of glucose
3. Fasting hypoglycemia

COMMON NEURO-LABS

Aldolase, CK, muscle Bx: myopathies. **B-12**: Peripheral neuropathy. **Check**: Folate +/- nerve BX.

RPR: Rule out exposure to syphilis. See neurosyphilis in the ID section.

TSH: **Check** thyroid for hyper/hypothyroidism.

Hypothyroid: Neurologic symptoms include changes in memory, cerebellar ataxia, muscle cramps, abnormal function of CN V, VII & VIII., prolonged relaxation phase of DTR.

Myxedema coma: Hypothyroidism: somnolence, slow mentation, subnormal temperature, hoarseness, muscle weakness then coma. **ESR**: erythrocyte sedimentation rate (see temporal arteritis section).

Lumbar Puncture: Oligoclonal bands: electrophoresis of CSF. Found in multiple sclerosis, inflammatory disease: syphilis, meningoencephalitis, subacute sclerosing panencephalitis & Guillain-Barré syndrome.

RADIOLOGY & TESTS

Carotid Arteriogram: Gold standard for diagnosis of vascular disease. Indications include TIA, CVA, and bleeds especially from aneurysm, **Disadvantage:** operator dependent in some cases not able to catheterize certain arteries, invasive procedure, risk of stroke (1:1000) & death. This procedure helps with precise location of the plaque; aids in identifying other causes of vascular disease (e.g., vasculitis, aneurysms), aids in the evaluation of existing & potential routes of collateral circulation. Other noninvasive methods include CT angiogram, MRA, and ultrasound.

Carotid endarterectomy (CEA): Indications include if stenosis > 70% & 6 weeks status post stroke or asymptomatic patient with high grade carotid stenosis of > 60%.

CT scan: Takes 72 hrs status post stroke to visualize on CT. If lesion is in the posterior fossa, may never see on CT. Use for: ischemic infarction, acute/chronic intracerebral subarachnoid hemorrhage, small-large ventricles, tumors, vascular malformations, abscess, bone lesions, calcifications.

Disadvantage: contrast reaction in contrast CT, check creatine prior to study especially with diabetics or patients using metformin, aminoglycoside & dehydrated patients.

Contrast CT vs. Non-contrast CT:

- **Contrast CT**: neoplasia, inflammation, vascular structures, AV malformation, hemangiomas, CNS infection, & intrinsic spinal cord lesions. Caution with patients that have allergies to iodine or shellfish, renal failure patients & patients on metformin. Avoid giving contrast to non-dialysis patients with creatine of > 1.5 mg/dl & hydrate patients (pre)post CT scan with normal saline. In emergency situations, most hospitals order a nonionic contrast study.

Prevention of contrast nephropathy:

1. **Fenoldopam** is used as an off label indication (i.e. not

FDA approved). Works on dopamine agonist receptors (DA- 1) to increase renal blood flow SE: liver failure, glaucoma.

2. Mucomyst: also used as an off-label to prevent contrast nephropathy.

- Non-contrast CT: indications include: hemorrhagic event, trauma, in suspected evolving stroke this is the initial study prior to anticoagulation to help exclude mass or bleed & helps with neuro-degenerative diseases.

CT angiograms: To examine carotid bifurcations & intracranial circulation.

Doppler: Accuracy (0-100%), tends to overestimate carotid stenosis.

Electroencephalography (EEG): Used in patient with changes in mental status, seizures, pseudoseizure metabolic encephalopathy, & Creutzfeldt-Jacob disease. EEG does not exclude epilepsy or focal pathology. Barbiturates can produce an isoelectric EEG.

Electronystagmography: Used to characterize nystagmus disturbances of eye movements that involve fast movements.

EMG: Direct test needle is placed in the belly of the muscle. **Check**: for nerve root problem & demyelination disease.

Lumbar Puncture Indications include rule out meningitis (infection), negative CT for subarachnoid hemorrhage, non-infectious inflammation (GBS, SLE), demyelinating disease & papilledema of unknown origin. Needle inserts at L4-L5: Passes: Skin, fascia, ligaments (supraspinous, interspinous, ligamentum flavum "pop," epidural space, dura mater, subdural space, arachnoid, subarachnoid space CSF. Do not pass Pia.

Tube 1: 2 ml for Protein & glucose. (obtain serum glucose).
Tube 2: 1-2 ml Gram stain & bacterial culture
Tube 3: 1-2 ml, Cell count & differential, serology
Tube 4: Cytology, stain acid fast, oligoclonal bands, serology, immunoglobulins.

Complications: Herniation, status post LP headache (give caffeine, lay patient down, or blood patch)

Contraindications: skin infection in the lumbar region, coagulation disorder, bleeding diathesis & ↑ ICP. It is important to analyze CSF immediately due to WBC lyses.

MRA (Magnetic Resonance Angiogram): Accuracy (0-100%). If 99% occluded & not sure if total occluded then order Doppler, together 95% accurate. Evaluate carotid arteries, IC vessels, circle of Willis, AV malformation, hemangiomas, aneurysms, TIA, strokes. **Advantage**: noninvasive, good screening tool for extra/intracranial vascular disease.
Disadvantages: technically demanding, may overestimate degree of vascular stenosis, may miss small vessel disease of < 3 cm.

MRI: +/- contrast agent: gadolinium has no risk for renal failure & allergies to agent are rare. MRI is the study of choice for most spinal imaging. It has better spatial & contrast resolution than CT; indications include soft tissue resolution, cancers patients with back pain & neurologic symptoms. Patients with neural claudications, demyelination, spinal, nerve root disease, pathology in the posterior area of brain & cisterns

Other advantages include the ability to see multiplanar images. Acute strokes are not seen on CT especially in the first 12 hours of stroke.

Disadvantages: time consuming, difficult for claustrophobic patients, not as sensitive as CT, or calcifications, hemorrhage, sensitive to movement (patient must hold very still).

Contraindication: Pacemaker & defibrillator devices, aneurysms clips.

Magnetic Resonance Spectroscopy: Identify chemical compounds (lactate) in the CNS used in Alzheimer, HIV, & Multiple sclerosis.

Myelograms: Used in patients with contraindications to MRI. Sensitive for disk pathology helps exclude cord compression in some cancer patients. Complications include CSF leak, meningitis & seizures.

Nerve Biopsy: use in the evaluation of inflammation disease (sarcoidosis) & infections (leprosy).

Nerve conduction velocity (NCV) study: The test uses surface electrodes to test motor or sensory: median, ulnar, radial, sural, saphenous, tibial, peroneal & lateral cutaneus nerve. It is useful in distinguishing demyelination that usually has decrease NCV from muscular disorder that has normal NCV with low amplitude.

PET scan: Positron emission tomography:
Check cerebral blood flow, brain metabolism, diffuse brain pathology, degenerative disease, dementia, cerebral blood flow & functional imaging.
Disadvantages: lower resolution than CT/MRI.

SPECT: **S**ingle **p**ositron **e**mission **c**omputerized **t**o**m**ography: seizure study, degenerative diseases advantages: sensitive for diffuse brain pathology, lower resolution than CT/MRI.

Ultrasound:

Advantages: easy to use, can be used in premature infants to rule out hemorrhage

Disadvantage: does not access vertebral arteries, less sensitive/ specific than MRA.

GENETICS

AUTOSOMAL DOMINANT: (AD) If female (Aa) heterozygous & female (AA) homozygous = 50% of children will express the disease.

AD : Alport syndrome (see CN VIII), Ehlers-Danlos syndrome & Marfan syndrome.

Huntington: 100% penetrance. (See Motor section).

Charcot-Marie-Tooth: Male > female it can also be an X-link or AR disease (other names include Peroneal muscular atrophy, Hereditary motor sensory neuropathy Type I children, Type II seen in adults) foot deformities Pes cavus, hammer toes, stork legs, gait changes, distal weakness & progressive wasting legs (muscle 87 atrophy), DTR decrease/absent, decrease vibration/pain/ temperature in stocking glove distribution.

Dx: Electromyography/nerve conduction study testing, sural nerve biopsy is rarely indicated

Rx: leg brace.

Myotonic dystrophy: Most common form of muscular dystrophy among Caucasians, adult onset, Chromosome 19, trinucleotide repeats of CTG in myotonin gene. Anticipation phenomenon: disease worsens with next generation.

S/s: worsen with cold temperature, "hatchet face" appearance due to temporalis, masseter, ptosis and facial muscle atrophy, weakness, low intelligence. Other symptoms include atrophy of sternomastoids, testicle & ovary; inability to release grip, myotonia can be elicited by percussion.

Check: EMG: myotonia, muscle biopsy, & other endocrinopathies. Death: myopathy, conduction defects & MVP.

Rx: symptomatic, braces for foot drop, Phenytoin & Pace maker.

Neurofibromatosis I (Von Recklinghausen): Chromosome 17q11.2 autosomal dominant, café-au-lait macules, axillary & inguinal freckling, Pre-puberty 5 or more lesions of 5 mm, if post-pubertal 6+ 15 mm. Lisch nodules, neurofibromas, acoustic neuroma, ↑ risk malignancy. *Ras* tumor-suppressor protein is associated with optic gliomas, meningiomas, pheochromocytomas, & CML.

Neurofibromatosis II: Chrom. **22, bi**lateral acoustic neuromas. Patients have increase frequency of meningiomas, spinal schwannomas & cataracts; Patients will have Café au lait spots with normal IQ.

(Z): Olivopontocerebellar: Atrophy: adult, onset cerebellar ataxia, dysarthria, extrapyramidal signs & symptoms.

(Z): Hypokalemic periodic paralysis: Defective calcium channels episodic paralyses due to stress, high carbohydrate diet, exercise, low potassium levels.

Two subtypes:

1. Familial autosomal dominant seen in adolescence
2. Hypokalemic periodic paralysis especially in Asians

Check TSH with this subtype; hyperthyroidism can produce hypokalemic periodic paralysis. Also, condition is associated with renal disease, alcohol, and steroids. Patient can have a provocative test: 50 to 100g oral glucose in order to illicit paralyses.

Rx: KCL, low-carbohydrate diet, & the carbonic anhydrase inhibitor.

Tuberous sclerosis: Chromosome 9: Seizures, infantile spasms, progressive psychomotor retardation, adenoma sebaceum (raised, red or yellow papules on the face), Shagreen patches (oval-shaped pigmented, smooth or crinkled, with firmer texture than normal skin appearing on the trunk or lower back), ash-leaf hypopigmentation, associated with Giant cell astrocytoma. Patients are at increase risk for renal cell carcinoma, angiomyolipoma & rhabdomyomas.

ddx of a patient with mental retardation + café au lait spots, should consider McCune-Albright or Tuberous sclerosis.

Von Hippel-Lindau syndrome: Hemoglobin & hematocrit elevated, retinal hemangioblastoma, spinal cord vascular malformations, polycystic kidney, pancreatic cysts, pheochromocytoma, patients at increased risk for renal cell carcinoma abnormality found on Chromosome 3p.

X-LINK: If Dad x-link recessive + mom (normal) = transmission to son = 0% but transmission to daughter is 100% will have disease but not express it.

(Z): Adrenoleukodystrophy: Patients have peroxisomal enzyme deficiency, rapid central demyelination, retinitis pigmentosa, seizures, spasticity, mental retardation & at increase risk of adrenal insufficiency that is unresponsive to ACTH.
Check: with MRI for demyelination.

Becker's: Milder than Duchenne still mobile at 40, but slow progression of disease & later onset of disease, IQ is normal. Low dystrophin levels due to abnormal dystrophin gene on Xp21.

Duchenne muscular dystrophy: Mutation of dystrophin gene, onset 1st decade of life; male: weakness of shoulder & pelvic girdle muscle, pseudohypertrophy gastrocnemii, difficulty with stairs, rising from floor, no myotonia, Gowers sign (climbs up on self to stand up) wheel chair bound by age 11.
Check: ↑ CPK, muscle Bx, absent dystrophin levels, EMG (small polyphasic potentials).Death is usually due to cardiomyopathy or restrictive pulmonary disease by age 25.
Rx: corticosteroids, physiotherapy.

Fragile-X: CGG (**C**ee **G**iant **G**onads) repeats, mental retardation, long thin face, large ears, & macroorchidism. The disease is seen in both female/male, male more severe disease than female.
Dx: direct DNA testing.

Lesch-Nyhan: Mutations in the gene coding for the enzyme hypoxanthine-guanine phosphoribosyltransferase (HPRT), which then causes increase Uric Acid levels; symptoms include mental retardation, self-mutilation, & gout.
Rx: allopurinol (block xanthine oxidase).

AUTOSOMAL RECESSIVE: (AR) If male (Aa) heterozygous + female (Aa) heterozygous then 1/4 will express the disease, ½ will be carriers & ¼ normal offspring.

(Z): Abetalipoproteinemia (Bassen-Kornzweig): Patients have absence of low-density beta-lipoprotein, low serum cholesterol & VLDL, acanthocytes in blood, retinal pigmentary degeneration, fat malabsorption, neuromuscular abnormalities, ataxia, & sensory motor neuropathy; autosomal recessive mutation on chrom 4q. **Rx**: supportive, Vitamin E & fat-soluble vitamins may improve neuropathy.

Ataxia-Telangiectasia: (AR) DNA repair defect (B & T cells), recurrent sino-pulmonary infection, telangiectasias seen typically in the nose, face, & neck. Other symptoms include cerebellar ataxia & at increase risk of having a malignancy (lymphomas and acute leukemias).
Check: elevation of serum alpha-fetoprotein level, IgA, IgG, defective gene in AT has been mapped to chromosome 11q22.3.

Faber's: Ceramidase defect: accumulation in nerves.

Friedreich ataxia: Most common hereditary ataxia, 3 long tracts degenerate: pyramidal, dorsal, spinocerebellar, optic atrophy, No DTR, ↑ Incidence of diabetes mellitus, most die of ♥ myopathy 90 (sinus sick syndrome, hypertrophic obstructive cardiomyopathy) before 40 year old. Autosomal recessive (AR) on Chromosome 9q13 (GAA-repeat expansion). The MRI may show atrophy. Patients are wheelchair bound from age 11-25; Most die between the ages of 30 and 40.

Gaucher's: Lacking glucocerebrosidase, increase glucosylceramide levels.

Hartnup's: Defect in tryptophan absorption.
S/s: similar to pellagra disease (Dermatitis, Dementia, Diarrhea and Death). Other symptoms include: cerbellar ataxia, & mental retardation.
Rx: Niacin

(Z): Krabbe (globoid cell leukodystrophy): Decrease β-glucocerebrosidase, loss of myelin, mental retardation, rapid spontaneous nystagmus globoid bodies & CSF ↑ protein.

McArdle: Deficit of glycogen phosphorylase: weakness, cramping after exercise.

Metachromatic leukodystrophy: Arylsulfatase A absent from urine and serum, increase sulfatides, increase forgetfulness, rapid deterioration, hepatosplenomegaly, dementia, ataxia, urine sulfatide test +. MRI: diffuse symmetrical demyelination.

(Z): Refsum: Defect: phytanic acid metabolism causes pigmentary retinal degeneration, progressive sensory motor neuropathy, cerebellar ataxia, sensorineural deafness, anosmia, bone defects, icthyosis, & cardiac conduction defects

(Z): Riley-day (familial dysautonomia)**:** Decrease pain & temperature sensation, decrease lacrimation, decrease patellar reflex, pupillary hypersensitivity to parasympathomimetic agents; Poor ANS control, autosomal recessive on 9 (q31–q33).

Phenylketonuria (PKU): Musty odor decrease phenylamine, increase tyrosine, mental retardation (MR) & cerebral myelin degeneration.

Galactosemia: Deficient in galactose-1-phosphate uridyl transferase causing mental retardation, cataracts & cirrhosis.

(Z): Werdnig-Hoffman: (see motor).

Wilson disease: AR, chromosome 13, hepatolenticular degeneration defect of copper metabolism leading to basal ganglion lesion, liver & psychiatric abnormalities (personality changes, dementia & depression). Kayser-Fleischer ring around cornea seen on slit lamp.
Neurologic S/s: ataxia, clumsiness, coarse tremor, spastic dystonia, cardiomyopathy & hypogonadism.
Dx: decrease serum ceruloplasmin, liver Bx & increase urine copper excretion. In women, an IUD with copper is contraindicated.
Rx:
1. **B6, Zinc** (decrease intestinal copper absorption), if allergic to
2. **D-Penicillamine** (SE: leukopenia, thrombocytopenia, metallic taste & proteinuria) then use
3. **Trientine**.

MITOCHODRIAL: Mitochondrial gene transferred from mother.

(Z): Kearns-Sayre: (chronic progressive external ophthalmoplegia, CPEO, with Ragged-Red Fibers) Rare neuromuscular disorder, seen prior to age 20, ptosis, retinitis pigmentosa, cardiac (heart blocks), myopathy, ataxia, & short stature.
Check: for endocrinopathies.

(Z): Leber hereditary optic neuropathy: Male, bilateral painless optic neuropathy, bilateral visual loss with central scotomas (blind spots) age of onset is variable but usually prior to the 3rd decade of life. Other symptoms include tremor, extrapyramidal syndrome, seizures, mental retardation. Biopsy shows abnormal mitochondria & defects in respiratory enzymes in mitochondria.

(Z): Leigh syndrome (subacute necrotizing encephalomyelopathy): Deficiency of cytochrome C oxidase (COX), decrease or absent thiamine pyrophosphate, developmental delay seizure, ataxia, optic atrophy, myoclonus, recurrent emesis.
Check: lactate: pyruvate ratio, MRI & DNA analysis.

(Z): Myoclonus epilepsy: With ragged red fibers (MERRF) syndrome: ataxia, dementia, sensorineural hearing loss, optic atrophy, cardiomyopathy, CT: cerebral & cerebellar atrophy, muscle biopsy: mitochondrial myopathy.
Rx: clonazepam, valproic acid.

VITAMIN DEFICIENCY & EXCESS

Vitamin A deficiency: Bitot's spots & night blindness.

Vitamin B-1: Dry beriberi (neuropathy, confusion, & encephalopathy), Wet Beriberi (cardiomegaly & prolong QT), Wernicke disease or Korsakoff disease; other manifestations include: CHF, decrease DTR, loss of vibration sense
Rx: vitamin B1 100 mg, increase foods white whole grains, lean pork, and legumes.

(Z): Strachan syndrome: Vitamin B1 (thiamine) deficiency causes: spinal ataxia, optic nerve atrophy & nerve deafness.

Vitamin B-3 (Niacin): Ataxic, seizures, delusion, depression, & pellagra symptoms: dementia, dermatitis, & diarrhea.

Vitamin B-6:

> **ddx**: malabsorption, drug induced (See INH).
>
> Common signs include: cutaneous mucosal symptoms: (cheilosis), CNS symptoms (paresthesias, seizures), ascending sensory polyneuropathy & anemia.
>
> **Rx**: underlying cause, vitamin B 6.
>
> **Excessive vitamin B 6** causes**:** sensory neuropathy**.**

B-12 (cobalamin) deficiency (subacute combined degeneration of the spinal cord): It is important to rule out malabsorption; the disease affects (usually spinal cord), brain, optic nerves (central vision) & peripheral nerves; typical presentations are patients with **p**ernicious anemia (rarely have normal hematocrit).

> **S/s**: general *weakness, paresthesias* tingling, "**p**ins & needles" Feet > hands. Gait: unsteady, stiff, weakness of legs, sphincter abnormal, loss of vibration sense, loss of superficial sensation, dementia, & **p**sychosis.
>
> **Check**: serum concentrations of methylmalonic acid & homocysteine levels are increased. **Important to note** that only homocysteine is elevated in folate deficiency (& has no neurologic deficits).
>
> **Rx**: Cyanocobalamin or hydroxocobalamin.

Vitamin B-12: Ddx nitric oxide abuse will cause B12 decrease levels, pernicious anemia: dementia, loss of position & vibration sense in lower extremity, paresthesia & psychosis.

Vitamin E: Loss of proprioception, vibration, areflexia, ataxia & myelopathy.

> **ddx**: absorption pathology, cystic fibrosis, abetalipoproteinemia & chronic cholestatic hepatobiliary disease.
>
> **Rx**: Vitamin E supplementation.

Excessive vitamin E causes: reversible myopathy.

NEUROLOGIC COMPLICATIONS OF SYSTEMIC DISEASES & MISCELLANEOUS

DDX IN GENERAL: If you have trouble thinking of a differential thing of **VITAMINS PICS**: Vascular, Infectious, Traumatic, Autoimmune, Metabolic, Idiopathic & degenerative, Neoplastic, Substance abuse & toxic Psychiatric, Inflammation, Congenital (genetic) & Structural.

Dermatomyositis/Polymyositis: Female>male ages 5-15 & 40-60, symmetrical proximal muscle weakness most common presenting sign, heliotrope rash (reddish–violaceous eruption on the upper eyelids) & knuckles (Gottron's papules).
Check: CK (10x normal levels), aldolase, LDH, ESR, muscle Bx is diagnostic, & EMG: low amplitude potential, polyphasic action potential. Patients at increase risk for malignancy that includes cervical, lung, ovarian, pancreatic, bladder, gastric carcinomas, & non-Hodgkin lymphoma.

Hemochromatosis: Autosomal recessive hereditary disease causes iron to be absorbed in excess.
S/s: include weakness, abdominal pain, hepatomegaly, increase skin pigmentation, testicular atrophy; neurologic symptoms include dementia, ataxia, headaches & personality changes.
Check: transferrin levels, serum ferritin & liver biopsy.
Rx: Phlebotomy, diet (decrease: Vitamin C, alcohol, beef), & if disease severe then use **Deferoxamine**. Complications include cirrhosis, diabetes, cardiomyopathy & hypogonadism.

Hepatic encephalopathy: Hepatic failure (cirrhosis) causing ammonia to increase which then causes GABA in CNS to increase; reversible neuropsychiatric abnormalities include: mental status changes, asterixis, coma, decerebrate posture & fetor hepaticus.
Check: for infections, electrolyte imbalance acute alcohol intoxication.
Rx:
1. Lactulose
2. Neomycin
3. Flagyl
4. Low protein diet.

(Z): Maple syrup disease: Inability to metabolize isoleucine, lysine, & valine. Patients have neurologic deficit of the CNS, mental retardation & death.

SIADH: (Drug induced by oxytocin, opiates, chlorpropamide) moderate hyponatremia can induce neurologic signs & symptoms (seizures, etc).

Chronic SIADH: Demeclocycline to block the effect of the ADH at the level of the kidney tubule on a chronic basis increase urine Osm > serum Osm.

Porphyria: Autosomal dominant, Peripheral nerve:
Motor S/s: 1st weakness of proximal UE > LE, seizures & abdominal pain. Urine turns orange-brown if left standing.
Rx: Hematin & high carbohydrate diet.

Thrombotic Thrombocytopenic Purpura TTP: Anemia, renal/hepatic disease, petechiae,
Neurologic S/s: confusion, delirium & seizures.

Whipple disease (*Trophermyma whippleii,* gram positive actinomycete*)*: Typically, middle age Caucasian male symptoms include: weight loss, diarrhea, malabsorption, GI bleeding, neurologic (dementia, confusion, gait ataxia, ophthalmoparesis); other symptoms include: uveitis, retinitis & arthropathy. **Dx**: by endoscopy with small bowel biopsy (containing macrophages staining positive with periodic acid-Schiff stain), & PCR. **Rx**: Bactrim for 1 year.

GREAT IMITATORS

SLE: Female>male need 4 of 11 criteria: Butterfly rash, Discoid rash, Photosensitivity, Oral ulcers, Arthritis, Serositis (Pericarditis), Renal disorder, Neurologic (seizure, psychosis), Hematologic, Immunologic (ANA, Anti-Sm), ANA, & Anti-SR protein antibody assay (new test).
Rx: steroids.

Syphilis: (see ID)

MEDICATIONS & NEURO SIDE EFFECTS

(Z): Acyclovir SE: Neurotoxic (delirium, tremors, seizures), headache.

(Z): Allopurinol SE: Subacute progressive neuropathy.

Amantadine SE: Hallucinations, headaches, confusion & ataxia.

Amiodarone SE: Incoordination, ataxia, optic neuritis, peripheral neuropathy, myopathy & hypothyroid. Cardiac arrhythmia: whorl-shaped pigmented deposits in the corneal epithelium. Deposits are dosing dependent & reversible once discontinue medications. Visual symptoms are rare.

Asparaginase/procarbazine SE: Encephalopathy, lethargy & confusion.

(Z): Benzodiazepine toxicity SE: Weakness, ataxia, coma, & respiration depression.

Cisplatin SE: Sensory ataxia continues for 3 months status post discontinuation of medication.

(Z): Chlorpromazine SE: Psychoactive. SE: produces punctate opacities in corneal epithelium on lens surface, after long-term use.

Corticosteroids SE: Long term use: posterior subcapsular cataracts.

Chloroquine SE: Use in treatment of Malaria, SE: Corneal deposits retinopathy, asymptomatic, produces glare & photophobia. Deposits regresses with dc of med. Drug induce retinal damage, insidious & irreversible. "Bull's eye macular lesion".

(Z): Cytisine + 5-flurouracil SE: Reversible cerebellar syndrome.

(Z): Dapsone SE: Motor deficit like ALS.

Didanosine ddI (Videx), D4T (Zerit), ddC (Hivid), & 3TC (lamivudine) **SE:** Peripheral neuropathy.

(Z): Diphenylhydantoin SE: Seizure medication SE: dose dependent: Cerebellar vestibular effects horizontal nystagmus in lateral gaze, **vertigo** nystagmus in upgaze. (Whatever direction you are looking will cause nystagmus in that direction). Other symptoms include: vertigo, ataxia, even diplopia with mild increases of blood levels of medication. Reversible if drug is discontinued.

Digitalis SE: Intoxication produces "blurry vision" or abnormal color vision (chromatopsia) appears yellow with overdose, also blue, red, brown, & green. White halos around dark objects, fatigue, & weakness.

Ethambutol SE: Optic neuritis, decrease visual acuity TB med, Side effect: dose related, 15mg/kg/day, 25 mg, 50mg optic neuropathy in 1%, 5%, 15% incidence respectively. Onset visual loss with in 1 month of initiating medication, recovery may take months after discontinuing medication, occasionally visual loss permanent.

HMG-CoA reductase inhibitors **SE:** necrotizing myopathy.

Isoniazid (INH) **SE:** Slurred speech, seizures, pleural effusions, sensory, & neuritis.
Rx: Vitamin B6.

Lithium, Demeclocycline & methoxyflurane SE: Diabetes insipidus.

Lindane SE: Neurotoxic especially in children.

Metronidazole SE: Paraesthesias, disulfiram reaction with ETOH, & cardiomyopathy.

Methotrexate SE: Neurotoxicity, & leukoencephalopathy.

(Z): Minocycline SE: Vestibulitis & blue-black depigmentation.

(Z): Nitric Oxide SE: Neuropathy, megaloblastic anemia 2nd to vitamin B-12 deficiency, numbness & paresthesia.

Neomycin/Kanamycin **SE:** Neuromuscular blockade, respiratory depression & Oto/nephrotoxic.

(Z): Nitrofurantoin SE: Neuropathies, hemolytic anemia in patient with G6PD deficiency.

(Z): Penicillamine SE: Drug induced myasthenia (ptosis, weakness).

Quinine SE: Cinchonism: tinnitus, headache, deafness, & shock.

Rifampin: Uveitis & red secretions (tears, urine, sweat).

(Z): Retinoids SE: Bone spurs that may pinch on nerve.

Sulfamethoxazole SE: Phototoxicity & kernicterus in infants.

(Z): Thioridazine SE: Pigmentary retinopathy, & cardiac toxic.

Vincristine SE: Peripheral neuropathy.

Zidovudine SE: Mitochondrial myopathy.

Myopathy SE: Colchicine, penicillamine, cocaine, & ETOH.

Neuropathies SE: Organophosphates, acrylamide & N-hexane.

Peripheral Neuropathies SE: Per-hexylene & thalidomide.

INTERNET SITES

Eye simulator: http://cim.ucdavis.edu/Eyes/Version1/eyesim.htm
Neurology online: http://www.neuropat.dote.hu/
Neuro exam: http://www.neuroexam.com/

Neurology review for the Non-Neurologist is currently available as a Kindle format (e-book) on Amazon.com.

INDEX